I0428372

Ebola Survival Kit

Ebola Survival Kit

Cleanse, detoxify, decalcify, purify, and protect your body from all forms of virus, bacteria, toxin,disease and infection.

J. Guinan Stevens
and
C. L. Carmen

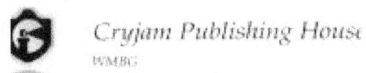 Cryjam Publishing House
WMBG

Ebola Survival Kit is available for download
in a digital format on Amazon.com
For more information, contact the publisher.

Published by Cryjam Publishing
Cryjampublishing.blogspot.com
cryjampub@gmail.com

Printed in the United States of America

To you, the reader

Contents

A note to the reader:

This book is not a cure or remedy for Ebola. It is a combination of very old holistic remedies. There is currently no official cure for Ebola. The FDA will not even allow the serum ZMapp to be called a cure. As of right now the only thing that can cure Ebola is the body's own immune defenses. The fit immune system has more chance of survival than the compromised immune system. We wrote this book to help you build the best immune system that you can have, and to stack the odds of survival in your favor. These methods will help protect against the Ebola threat. They also work for many other viral and bacterial pathogens.

C. L. Carmen and J. Guinan Stevens are neither doctors nor healthcare workers. Recently however we have discovered the perfect combination of preventative, easy to do practices that will transform your body and life. This combination of routines has transformed our bodies and immunity in just a few weeks.

The youngest of these modes is over a century old. Another has been in use for a thousand years. Whilst, the oldest dates back four millennia. These techniques have been applied generationally throughout different parts of the world. When done properly these means are all safe and highly effective. When you combine them all the results are nothing short of miraculous. This program will greatly increase your immunity.

Ebola is a threat that looms on the horizon. As are the viral and bacterial pathogens that we face everyday. There has never been a better time to improve your immunity. We can do this together, and by doing so we will change the world for the better. Imagine if world wide we all raised our level of health together. Through this program we will will banish aches and pains. We will eradicate so much sickness and suffering. We will be prepared for the Ebola threat and any subsequent menaces that

mother nature throws our way. We ask you to join in our crusade to be the best, healthiest, happiest person that you can be. We know that all who embark on this journey will be amazed at the astounding transformation within just a few short weeks. You will be awed by the person you become. You will completely forget all the aches, pains, and complaints that you have right now.

1. What is a Virus and What is Ebola*

[1]*"Viruses are capsules with genetic material inside. They are very tiny, much smaller than bacteria. Viruses cause familiar infectious diseases such as the common cold, flu and warts. They also cause severe illnesses such as HIV/AIDS, smallpox and hemorrhagic fevers. Viruses are like hijackers. They invade living, normal cells and use those cells to multiply and produce other viruses like themselves. This eventually kills the cells, which can make you sick."* Viruses are organisms that do not respond to antibiotics, therefore you must treat the symptoms. Your immune system has to be working at its optimal capacity, so that it can kick out those hijackers and allow your body to function normally. Ebola is a virus that is transmitted from human to human via bodily fluids. It is not transmitted through the air. It is not a waterborne illness. To catch Ebola you have to be directly exposed to a person who is a carrier and they have to be displaying symptoms of the disease. According to the CDC symptoms usually appear anywhere from two to twenty-one days after exposure, with eight to ten days being the median for when symptoms start to appear. The symptoms of Ebola are fever, headache, joint aches, muscle aches, weakness, diarrhea, vomiting, stomach pain, lack of appetite, and abdominal bleeding. Soon after the hemorrhagic fever starts producing caustic symptoms. Those are terrible things that we do not want anyone to suffer. Please bear with us as we talk about the history of Ebola. We will soon disclose how you can protect yourself, and everyone that you love, from disease in general.

In 1976, Ebola (named after the Ebola River in Zaire) originated in Sudan and Zaire. The first outbreak of Ebola (Ebola-Sudan) infected over 284 people, with a mortality rate

---

[1]. Definition taken from the NIH: National Institute of Allergy and Infectious Diseases website.

of 53%. A few months later, the second Ebola virus emerged
from Yambuku, Zaire, Ebola-Zaire (EBOZ); it had the highest
mortality rate of any eruption (88%), and infected 318 people.
That year marks the second worst scourge of Ebola with 602
reported cases and 431 fatalities. As of early August 2014
Guinea, Sierra Leone, Liberia,and Nigeria had a combined case
count of 1,322 souls suffering from Ebola; 718 of the infected
people had passed away at that point. There had been 3,069
reported cases with 1,552 deaths by August, 28, 2014. The
World Health organization announced on September third that
the death toll had risen to at least 1900 people with over 3500
people infected. That is a 54.28% mortality rate. This is
currently the worst paroxysm of Ebola that the world has ever
seen. It is disturbing when you compare the numbers between
early August and late August. 40% of the total cases were
reported in the last three weeks in August. The World Health
Organization has warned that there could be as many as 20,000
people infected before the outbreak can be brought under
control. WHO announced a road map in late August
to manage this catastrophe. The objective is to stop
transmission of the virus within the next six to nine months.
The road map also seeks to improve international response
while addressing the social-economic problems that this plague
has caused. More people have died in the 2014 Ebola outbreak
than all other flare-ups combined over the past 40 years. As of
October 1st there have been 6,500 confirmed cases resulting in
more than 3000 deaths. The outbreak continues to grow
exponentially. The United States now has confirmed it's first
case in Dallas, Texas. A Liberian man who came to the U.S.
unknowingly was infected. He is being treated at Texas
Presbyterian Hospital. Whether he infected anyone else is
currently unknown. On Friday September 27 Dr. Tom Frieden,
Director of the CDC addressed world health officials. He said,

'the outbreak in West africa was a test," and that, " we the World, failed this test." The CDC has predicted that 1.4 million people could be infected by January 2015. This situation is definitely out of control, it is a tragedy unfolding before us all. The numbers are accelerating at an alarming rate, and will most likely continue to do so until this pandemic can be restrained.

Let us take a quick look at ZMapp. The whole world is hoping that this serum is the cure. Financial markets are abuzz about this opportunity, so what is ZMapp? ZMapp is a serum for Ebola. It is not a vaccine and it certainly is not a government approved cure. Our understanding is that it is a blend of genetically engineered Ebola antibodies. The goal is that it will help boost the patients' immunity to fight off the virus. Zmapp is actually two different serums from two different companies combined together. The San Diego based Mapp Biopharmaceutical created MB-003. A Canadian company Defyrus inc. has made Zmab. LeafBio, a part of Mapp Biopharmaceutical acquired the licenses and combined the two serums in hopes that two would be stronger than one. MB-003 was created by injecting mice with Ebola and extracting antibodies. Mouse antibodies do not work in humans so they built in human DNA to make chimera antibodies that are compatible with humans. Interestingly enough the company is using an Australian tobacco plant to grow the antibodies. When they tested MB-003 on monkeys one or two days after infection they had a 43% survival rate. The Canadian Zmab has three types of mice Ebola antibodies as well. When they tested Zmab on monkeys 100 % survived when injected 24 hours after exposure. 50% survived when treated 48 hours after exposure. In Humans, symptoms appear two to twenty one days after exposure. Humans are not monkeys, we are close, but not the same. Most of those who were infected did not know that they had contracted the virus on the second day.

What is the drug's success twenty one days after exposure? A form of early detection would be of great benefit to ensure this drug's success. Leafbio who acquired the licenses for both serums has made ZMapp. ZMapp is a combination of the two serums. To our knowledge it still has not gone through any official human clinical trials. The FDA requires many stages of human trials which could take years. The two Americans who were infected in Liberia and brought to Atlanta were treated with ZMapp. Both of them survived. As of early September 2014 it had been reported that seven people had been officially treated with ZMapp. Of those seven people, two have unfortunately died. That is a 28.57% mortality rate. The drug has greatly increased the chances of survival in that group of patients. Zmapp gives us all hope, and we applaud the scientists who are working so hard to cure this horrible disease.

The cure for Ebola is still very far off, as of now Leafbio has a limited supply of the drug; and even if they had great quantities it still has not been thoroughly tested for safety. We suspect that part of the problem on the supply side is that you have to grow a tobacco crop each time you make the drug. This is our simple understanding of the drug's approach: to introduce multiple types of fabricated Ebola antibodies into the patient which will assist the immune system and speed up natural recovery. In the last week of August 2014 ZMapp achieved some amazing breakthroughs. In a clinical trial, ZMapp was able to heal 18 monkeys that were infected with the Ebola virus. The study was published online Friday August 29, 2014 in the medical journal Nature. The monkeys were treated with ZMapp three to five days after they were infected. This is further out than any other trail. This test was a complete success. Another trial used a different version of Zmapp and was just as successful. These studies have shown great promise. ZMapp still needs human clinical trials to determine the proper dose among other things. Mapp Biopharmaceuticals has announced that it could take several months to make the next Batch. ZMapp is being made in a plant in Kentucky that can make 20 to 40 doses in a month.

Our system of survival differs in that it focuses on naturally building your immune system so that it recognizes threats and can start fighting them right away. We are hoping that this will increase the survival rate for people on the program. Ideally however this strategy is a flotation device to prevent drowning. ZMapp when it is approved will be the boat that scoops you out of the water and deposits you safely on land. Our program's objective is to get your immunity in shape so you can tread water easily with your life preserver and wait for rescue. When the rescue boat will arrive we do not know. We want you to be able to survive as long as you can and possibly have the strength to swim ashore. When your life is in peril do not take it for granted that you will be rescued. You have
to be ready to save yourself. We want your immunity to be in great shape and trust us the makers of ZMapp want the same thing. Infected people with stronger immunities will respond to ZMapp much more positively than people with compromised immunities.

This virus scares us, it has frightened us so much that it has motivated us to get our message out. In this day and age you have to be as strong as you can not only physically, but mentally and spiritually as well. We live in a time of modern miracles both medical and otherwise. This thaumaturgy comes at a drastic cost. We currently have the highest life expectancy of all time and are blessed with very advanced healthcare. We also live in more comfort than ever thanks to technology. There has never been a better time to be alive than right now but modern science has its limits. There are many people suffering from viruses that can be managed but a true cure still eludes us. Herpes, HPV, and HIV just to name a few. Antibiotics have been a modern Godsend, but they also have their limits. Societies' over prescription and use, paired with a food supply that is laden with antibiotics has caused a growing problem;they do not work as well as they used to. There are bacterial infections now that are extremely resistant to antibiotics. Even though science is quite advanced, our current medical system is very limited in some ways. It seems we have become a society that takes prescription medication to manage the symptoms of our illnesses, but when it comes to curing these same illnesses we are not quite as good. Amidst all our modern medical miracles we still cannot cure the common cold.

The age of comfort in which we all live comes at a price in the form of pollution and stress. We are currently bombarded with pollution and toxins in our environment that seriously compromise our immune systems. There has never been a time when the life
expectancy was more; however, we are breathing, eating, and drinking in toxins at record levels. So yes you are likely to live a long life, but we cannot promise how great you are going to feel. We do not accept that, we believe there is something you can do.

Earlier we stated the only way to cure most viruses is for your immune system to fight them off. In that case we better make our immune systems as impregnable as they can be. That is exactly what we plan to do. We are going to lay out a multi-prong approach that is going to make you stronger and revive you mentally, physically and spiritually. When you employ our techniques and make them part of your daily routine you will start to experience miracles of your own. All the side benefits of this program are wonderful, but the main goal of this book is to strengthen your immune system. That way you will be prepared and ready in the unfortunate event that we do have to deal with Ebola or something like it. Hopefully Ebola will never be a problem for most of us. However, the problem that is prepared for is much easier to deal with than the problem that is ignored.

Ebola survival kit will prepare and protect you in the event of a worst case scenario. As an added benefit you will enjoy healing current conditions and preventing future conditions. Join us in becoming the strongest, healthiest people that we can be. It is not going to be easy, but a little bit of effort goes a long way. You can do it! This survival kit is a jump start manual to supercharging your immune system. We want you to prepare and protect now. There is a plethora of information available on all the methods mentioned in this book. We encourage you to do your own research and make your own decision. The purpose of this book is to quickly learn what you should be doing so that you can start as soon as possible.

This program is an economical no nonsense way of getting healthy. The program consists of Eight pillars of protection for your immune system. Each pillar is simple, it often boils down to being more mindful of your choices when it comes to that aspect of your life; for example always use what you have and replace the staples of your life with the best ingredients that you are able to. Try not to waste and make choices that are wise instead of based on impulses. That being said let us delve into the pillars themselves.

The first Pillar of protection has to to with the mind. The first thing that has to change in your life is your mental perception. Negativity blocks us, not just emotionally but physically and spiritually as well. The first step in becoming a healthy person is to change your paradigm. Once the mind starts to change the body will follow. You will find yourself not wanting to harm yourself or anyone else. Naturally as you become more mindful you will find that your eating habits will start to change. Which leads us to the second pillar of the program... Diet. The old saying, *"you are what you eat from your head down to your feet,"* is true: if you want to be a healthy super strong person you must ingest super foods. It is exactly like Popeye and his spinach. Which leads us to the third pillar... exercise. A positive mind coupled with a properly nourished body gives you the energy to build a body that reflects all the change happening on the inside. We are not talking about running marathons, unless that is your dream. We are talking about simple life changes, about getting up and active. Every little bit helps. Once your mind is working positively, you are being mindful of what you eat, and you start strengthening your body through exercise you are ready for the fourth pillar of the program... Supplementation.

Supplementation is very important these days. Eat all the calories you like, we doubt that you will get all the vitamins that your body needs to function properly. This pillar requires the use of daily vitamin supplements to strengthen you on a cellular level. Which bring us to the fifth pillar of the program....the Oxygen Cleanse. You are going to cleanse your body of all past infections while strengthening your immune and cardiovascular system. This is all done with an affordable, safe easy to do home therapy. You will have the power of oxygen working for you. This brings us to the sixth pillar of the program. Which is lacto fermentation. Now that you are thinking positively, eating mindfully, living an active lifestyle, supplementing your diet, and purifying your entire system it is time to take your diet to the next level. This is fermentation. It is easy, cost effective, preserves food, and is just plain delicious. Not to mention the fact that it helps to supercharge your immune system. The seventh pillar of the program is to cleanse the sinus and oral cavities. These are the places where we are most likely to catch bugs and viruses: ears, nose, throat, mouth and eyes. So it is imperative to have this system functioning at peak performance. This brings us to the Eighth and final pillar of the program.... Kvass. Kvass is the second of our miracle elixirs, the first being the Oxygen Cleanse. Beet Kvass is simple to make and incredibly nourishing. Now that you know what you are in for its time to take a more in depth look at each of the pillars independently. This program is uncomplicated, if we can do this anyone can. Failure is not trying in the first place. Your journey to absolute health and resistance to disease begins now.

3.The Mind

Our brain is our best friend and our worst enemy. Like the yin-yang, it must be in balance. To attain that balance it must be clean, so that clarity and ease can be attained. With ease comes health and happiness. We must banish the dis-ease from our minds to ensure a clear pathway to ultimate health. In order to do this you must empty your mind of all negativity past and present. You must learn to forgive yourself for your perceived past mistakes and learn to truly forgive others. You cannot spend anytime on a,"what if,";or an, "I should have,"; or even a, " I cannot believe that they did that to me." The past is gone and there is nothing that you can do to bring it back, nothing at all. Woulda, coulda, shouldas are not allowed. Let it all go resolutely. Do it for real! Forgive yourself and stop punishing yourself. You deserve to live and be the healthiest you that you can be. It is okay to be happy with who you are and what your circumstances are. Stop comparing yourself to everyone else. The only marker for your yardstick is you. How much do you want to grow? You at this moment are the best you that you can be. You also have the opportunity at this very moment to become the person of your dreams. You can become whatever or whomever you desire starting right now. As you forgive others that have hurt, belittled, or done you wrong, no matter how bad, you will start to build spiritual strength. As you forgive these people and release them from your thoughts you will be getting rid of massive amounts of oppressive negativity. This process is long and on going. Your subconscious mind has been feeding on negativity in connection with these people and events for a long time. So you have to accept that it is going to take a sustained effort on your part. You cannot change negative thought patterns overnight or even in a week. It requires commitment to flood your mind with positive thoughts of forgiveness toward others and most importantly yourself. We are our own worst critics, and for most of us no one is harder on us than ourselves. We have experienced all the offenses, rejections, disappointments, injuries, and worst of all failures. We have been there and been first hand witnesses to all our mistakes, failures, and bad decisions. The worst of all these is when we let ourselves down, when we lie to ourselves, and injure ourselves both mentally and physically. The human condition is to have all these things and worse thrown at you. Life is very hard. Interacting with people professionally and socially is very difficult. Living in our own skins and interacting with ourselves can be arduous. As humans we are naturally judgmental. We judge things. Which piece of fruit is better. We also judge other people and ourselves, often negatively. It is just a natural tendency in today's society to have a negative spin on everything. To be super healthy we need to flood our minds with loving thoughts of forgiveness and good will towards others and most importantly ourselves. The old saying forgive and forget is more challenging to do than it sounds. We have all experienced people being extremely awful and doing horrible things to us, they inflict injuries that do not go away overnight. But slowly over time you will gain the power to let it all go and when you do, what a glorious happy day it will be. Positive thought is a very powerful thing. The problem is that society overwhelms us with negative imagery and thoughts through our media and entertainment. When negative thoughts rule the mind it is dis-eased, not at ease. When you consciously input positive, loving thoughts of forgiveness you are slowly putting your mind at ease and entering a healthy state. Once you have begun the process of forgiveness it is time to take it to the next level. You have to release all pettiness and jealousy from your life. It is by no means easy, but the rewards are definitely worth the effort. Release the negative thoughts and comparisons to others and you will reap the benefits of a healthy mind that will help you attain whatever goals you desire in life. Now that we are feeding healthy positive thoughts into our minds we are ready to move to the last step of mind for our purpose. That is gratitude. Gratitude is one of the most powerful emotions that we experience in life. It is right up there with love. It is interesting to note that negative hurtful emotions such as anger and hate are far easier to produce than the higher more powerful emotions of love and forgiveness. The more we can be grateful and experience that emotion, the stronger our mind and spirit becomes. As humans we always look at what we do not have. We focus on our wants, desires and what we lack. This floods our psyches with negativity and we become focused on lack, want, and what we do not have. As our conscious thoughts are feeding this lack into our subconscious, we are actually doing ourselves great harm. Because our subconscious does not judge it just listens and reacts. If you give it negative thoughts of what you lack that is exactly what your subconscious will reproduce in your life and experiences in this world. If you consciously input thoughts of love, forgiveness,empathy, and gratitude(all the highest of emotions), that is exactly what your subconscious will manifest in your life and experiences.

Let us tell you a little story: last night C. L. was about to go out for a jog. Just before she headed out the door she said " It is fantastic not to feel any pain in my ankle," as it had been injured a week earlier. As C. L. walked down to the jogging path she
stumbled over the edge of the pavement twisting her ankle. Right then she had an epiphany that her subconscious had given her exactly what it thought that she wanted. C. L. thought she was being positive and sending herself a positive message but her syntax was wrong. The subconscious does not understand negatives. The subconscious heard "It is fantastic to feel any pain in my ankle." She manifested exactly that within seconds of thinking it. She should have said something like, "my ankle feels great," and left it like that. Words and thoughts are very powerful, we have to use both judiciously.

As you gain power over your own thoughts and transform your mind into a powerhouse of positivity you will be amazed to see how quick the body follows. A healthy mind and body can fight off virus, bacteria and toxins. A healthy mind and body is ready to survive even the worst circumstances. There are many ways to achieve loving, positive, forgiving, grateful thoughts. Here are some traditional and not so traditional methods that can help get your mind in a healthy state.

The most traditional method is through meditation, reflection, and actually placing affirmative thoughts in your mind. This is easy, completely free, and does not take that much time. The result is not instant, it is cumulative. The more you focus on positivity, the more you remove negativity and sickness from your mind. It is an ongoing pursuit that takes commitment. A few brief affirmations at the end of this chapter will be included if this is one of the courses you pursue.

Another traditional method to getting rid of negativity would be therapy, or psychiatric care. Psychiatrists and therapists have been helping people put there mind at ease for generations. I would
caution however against the prescription of psychoactive drugs. These defeat the whole purpose of this book. We are trying to make you healthy on a cellular level so that you are highly resistant to viral infection, not put you on a new drug that could possibly compromise your immune system and overall health. If you are already on medication you can do the program, but check with your doctor first. However there are many psychiatrists and therapists who do not rely on drugs to solve problems. They actually work through your problems and issues. Therapy can be a wonderful and freeing process that can definitely put your mind at ease. There are only two downsides. Therapy can be a very long and drawn out process. Therapy also is probably the most expensive option.

Another option is Hypnotherapy. Whether with an actual hypnotherapist or from a download hypnotherapy is very effective. When you see a hypnotherapist they make a recording of your session that you can listen to while relaxing every day. You can also download or buy recordings to be hypnotized at your leisure. Hypnotherapists can be quite expensive, but highly effective over time. Downloads and recordings are very affordable and in our opinion just as effective. hypnotherapy can be affordable, but it also takes a long term commitment to get full results. What we have found to be the most cost effective and gratifying are subliminals, binaural beats, and audio entrainment. By simply going onto youtube.com and performing a simple search of the above key words you will open up a world of possibilities. You will have a lot of choices but stay focused and listen to the ones that are going to help you with your goal of getting your mind in order. We have found that they are very effective to listen during our daily commute to and from work on the subway. Never ever listen to binaural

beats, hypnosis, or do any sort of entrainment while driving or operating any sort of motor vehicle. Those are a couple of options to help cleanse your mind of negativity and strengthen your brain and overall health. As your mind becomes positively charged it will take a natural interest in your overall health. The next steps in the process will happen almost automatically.

We have included a few positive affirmations which will help accelerate the process. We take a spiritually neutral tone with with these affirmations. We encourage you to personalize them for yourself. They can be changed to fit your personal religious or spiritual beliefs. The main thing is that you believe in something higher than yourself even if it is the Laws of Physics, or your subconscious.

Affirmation of forgiveness:

I know that the power of the universe flows through me as forgiveness. I forgive all those that have hurt me, done me wrong, or led me astray. I forgive you all and release you to the universe. I forgive anyone who has offended me today. I forgive myself for the negative thoughts and actions that I have had, and for any negative or hurtful thoughts that I have had today. I firmly resolve to have positive, constructive thoughts of love. My thoughts are always onwards and upwards.

Affirmation of gratitude:
I know that the power of the universe flows through me as gratitude. I am grateful for all the blessings that the universe has bestowed upon me. I am grateful for my health, my family, my friends, my career, and even my wonderful possessions. I am so lucky for everything I have. I am thankful for all the wonderful blessings and treasures that the universe is going to bestow upon me. I am truly thankful that all my goals are being achieved successfully. Thank you very much.

Affirmation of health:

I know that the power of the universe flows through me as universal healing power. Universal healing power flows through me eliminating everything unlike itself. I am healing and being regenerated on a cellular level. My body is in perfect health and immune to all infection, viruses, bacteria, toxins and parasites. I give thanks for my perfect health. Thank you.

Affirmation for universal well being:
I know that I am the physical expression of the power of the universe. I know that universal power manifests itself within in me as health, happiness, abundance, joy and love.

Repeat these affirmations in comfort and silence two to three times per day and you will have amazing results within a week or two.

Get your mind under control, you are in charge of it. Make it manifest what you truly want in your life. When you control your thoughts everything else in life seems to fall into place. As your brain
becomes healthier you will find yourself making better decisions automatically, which then leads us to our second pillar.

4. Diet

Diet is one of the most important things you can change to strengthen your immune system. This is not a book about weight loss. This is a book about making small changes in your life immediately that will cumulatively transform your immunity. This book is a crash course which will give your mind, body, and spirit the ability fight off viruses, bacteria, disease, toxins, parasites, and fungus. This is a book that prepares you for the worst case scenario, a world Ebola pandemic. We pray along with the rest of you that it never happens. Heaven forbid if it does spread to more countries, we want everyone around the world to be prepared as best they can. There is no miracle cure for Ebola. Just good old fashioned hydration and prayer as far as we have been able to find out. We implore you please make these changes in your life and by all means research into all of this on your own, but please do it quickly. We believe that if you make these changes to your life that you will be able to give yourself a fighting chance for survival. We know that the odds for survival will be much better for someone who is on this program. If we all do this together as a world community we will be prepared, and in a much healthier state than our current condition.

Diet is very hard for most people. We either do not care about it and let ourselves go, or we go to the other extreme and over control our diets and often develop illnesses of the mind and body. For the purpose of this book we want you to make a mindful effort to make healthy choices in your diet. We want you to be well nourished and happy. In our current world civilization and world economic markets we have let the genie out of the bottle when it

comes to food. In many countries in the world, the United
States for example, we have access to affordable empty
calories. If you
have a dollar in your pocket you can go to McDonald's get a
Mcdouble, and get a penny back! That is 390 calories right
there. If you have another buck in your pocket they have some
sort of soda deal, where you can get as many refills as you
want. Soda is cheap access to calories. We have been there,
seen it, and unfortunately done it many times in the past. The
most affordable calories in the United States are the
unhealthiest. They are all the ones that you can get coupons
for. If you are poor in the U.S. the least healthy food is exactly
what you have access to because it is the most affordable. Now
what if you are not poor and you invest in the best brands and
buy your foods from high end grocery stores? We do not
believe that the rich are in a better position when it comes to
healthy diets. In the U.S. we currently are experiencing a food
disaster. Our diets as a whole are terrible. We are the most
obese nation in the world. According to the Monday,
September 8, 2014 issue of Time Magazine by 2048 100% of
Americans will be obese. Diabetes, heart disease, and obesity
are just a few of the ailments that are growing rampantly. In the
U.S. we are literally eating ourselves to death. If your diet is
compromised, your immune system is also at risk. We do not
expect you to transform your whole diet over night, but we do
expect you to be conscious of what you eat. We also expect
you to try to make healthier choices from this point forward.

When you are first confronting your diet do not throw
away what is in your cabinet or your fridge. Read the label
before you prepare it, look at the portion size and adhere to it.
The first step in controlling your diet is to actually know what

you are eating and how much of your caloric intake for the day you are using up. We found a really great free app that we use religiously it is called *My Fitness Pal.* It tabulates everything for you and is quite easy to use. It has become an invaluable tool. Eat what you have until it is gone and then replace it with higher quality nutrient rich foods. We found ourselves craving lots of carbohydrates in the beginning. That precipitated feelings of deprivation, which allowed us to rationalize the buying of chips and gobbling them up. What we learned was do not deprive yourself of anything, just pay attention to the portion size. If you want chips eat them but do it responsibly.

Your body needs to be tamed just like your mind. When we spend a lifetime filling our bodies with caffeine, sugars, empty carbohydrates, and fat, we have to then ease it off gently. If you try to quit cold turkey you are asking for failure. Take your time and gently come off of the over processed foods. Always remember to restock with natural or organic alternatives. Start cooking quality nourishing simple meals. For example instead of buying Hamburger or Tuna Helper make your own, it is not much harder than making the box version.

Easy *Pasta Meal Recipe*

1 cup of dried pasta per serving that you want to make

Ground Beef,Ground Turkey, or Tuna (Keep in mind that the standard portion size for meat is 4 ounces)

whatever veggies you have on hand peas, carrots, onions, broccoli, whatever.

Bring your pasta water to boil in a large pot add the pasta.

In a saute pan brown your beef or turkey drain and set aside.

Clean and prep your veggies, if they are left overs and already cooked just set aside.

Drain your pasta and run under cold water
return it to the pot add the meat and veggies and mix. Add milk,cream,or soy milk. Combine
all ingredients, including any seasonings that you like. We put Bragg's liquid aminos in everything it takes away the need for salt. If you want to add butter feel free but remember to look at the standard portion. Put in a warm oven and bake at 350 until the milk starts to bubble which should be in about 15 minutes. Serve with your favorite salad and you have a complete meal free from artificial preservatives
and ridiculous amounts of salt.

We used to be the household that scoured the weekly grocery circulars looking for the best deals on Sodas that we could find. Three twelve packs for $ 8.00 was brilliant, Five for $10.00 was even better. We felt elated when we looked in our fridge, and it was stocked with our weekly haul and then one day it just happened. Suddenly the hard core Cola was being swapped out for Diet versions. It was a natural transition. It happened and we did not fight it. Listen to your body when it tells you that it is okay to change. Over time we stopped going to the grocery store every week looking for the best soda deal because we had gobs of it at home in the fridge unopened. Hmm... something was going on and then we realized that we did not need the soda anymore. Naturally we started replacing soda with water. One day we brewed some green tea. We put it in a pitcher,stuck it in the fridge, and to our surprise it was delicious. Your body will automatically adjust itself to your healthier eating habits. We are all addicted to the additives in our food. It is up to us as adults to break the cycle of addiction and to teach our children how to eat responsibly. There is an old saying," *eat to live don't live to eat."* We are asking everyone that lives in the world to embrace that mantra.

Medical science can do a plethora of things, but you only get one body. One temple to worship the benevolent God that you are becoming. Your mind is becoming more settled and your body is being nurtured from the inside. You should be feeling much more in control of everything. That is because you are freeing yourself from the shackles of negativity, the chains that bound you to eat from a place of emotional need. Which was a place of illusionary comfort rather than of sustenance. Stick with it, you are going to feel exceptional.

Become as healthy as you can no matter what your economic circumstances are. If vegetables are on sale purchase as many as you can. It is quite simple to make your own frozen veggies. Simply blanche (dip them for a few moments in boiling water), then remove the vegetables from the water, and place in a large bowl to cool. When you can handle them without burning yourself put standard servings into a freezer bag, remove all the air and put in the freezer. If you have enough variety make mixes just like they do in the store, let your imagination loose and have fun. If you can afford to buy a cry o-vac machine do it. If you want to eat red meat do it by all means. You should make the decision to eat less but of a higher quality and remember portion size. Save your colon some work, it is essential for the digestive system. It is in your digestive track that good health must flourish in order for you to live in ultimate health.

We must also pay attention to kitchen safety because hopefully you are spending more time in it. Be sure that all of your knives are sharp, a dull knife is an accident waiting to happen. It is vital that all of your surfaces are clean and that you wash all of your fruits vegetables and meats. Parasites and bacteria are not welcome in our healing bodies. At this point you have begun to work on the mind and the energy that fuels your body. Now it is time to burn some of that fuel. You are ready for the third pillar in the program.

So far we are improving the thoughts that we are putting into our minds, and what we are nourishing ourselves with. Addressing these two things alone will greatly increase your health and immunity. Now it is time to step up to the next level with exercise. We do not expect you to rush out the door and join the most expensive gym. We do not expect you to attain the services of a personal trainer. We expect you to try to become more active. We want you to pursue exercise, and athletic endeavors safely. That being said, personal trainers are certified professionals and gyms are usually run by dedicated fitness professionals. These people change lives every day and help people achieve their fitness goals. If you have the financial means a gym, personal trainer, or both might be the perfect solution. We have been members of gyms in the past and have had great results. Gyms and trainers require commitment and dedication, but they are not the only option.

The only thing you need to get into better shape is the body you are born with. Hopefully you have some clothes that would be appropriate to work out in, but if you do not, just use what you have. A nice pair of running or walking shoes would be ideal, but if that is not an option for you right now, use what you have. We just want to get you up and moving more than you are now. If you sit in a chair or on the couch all day, we want you to get out in the sun and go for a short walk. When that is easy for you maybe you will want to go for a short walk in the evening after dinner. After a while those short walks will become longer walks and you will be well on your way to fitness, health, and immunity. If you live a more active lifestyle, we want you to push your limits. Those with active careers and lifestyles need to realize that working is not enough to keep you in shape particularly as you age into your mid 30's and beyond. You have to push your limits. You need to find time for a simple exercise regime, if you can walk, then walk; if you can jog, then jog; if you can run, then run. Getting outside and moving around is so good for your mind, body, and soul. The urge to exercise is a natural progression that is the result of your work on your mind and diet. They all work together wonderfully to raise the level of your health. When you bring your health to a better state, you bring your immunity to a better state.

We told you in the last chapter about an app for smart phones that helps you manage your diet. There are also many free apps that will help you exercise. The incredible thing about these apps is that they connect to myfitnesspal and inform them of the calories you have burned during your workouts. That way you can manage your diet and get a complete picture of what is going on. When it comes to ways to get fit for free the smart phone, tablet, or computer are definitely the best way to do it. These apps are modern technological blessings. There has never been a time before when you could manage your diet, be physically trained, and log all of your activity for free. Smart phones and apps have really made gyms and personal trainers a thing of the past. Why pay money to a gym, and trainer; put money into gas, or public transportation; and take time out of your busy schedule to commute to the work out? Why would we do that when it is all on our phone for free? Maybe the apps are not as good as a personal trainer, but they are free and you have your phone with you wherever you go. With these apps you can do your work out at your level and pace anywhere in the world. You can even complete these exercises in a hotel room or bedroom. Our favorite programs are runkeeper for walking and jogging, and fitstar for short intense workouts you can do anywhere. We only use the free versions, the free versions of these apps are all you will ever need. They even work with heart rate monitors.

You are now flooding your mind with positive thoughts, improving your diet, exercising more, and tracking it all on your
smartphone. You are now employing three of the pillars of the program, but strong foundations are not built on three pillars. Now it is time complete the foundation.

6.Supplements

Vitamins and minerals are essential for building your super body. Now that you have started charting everything that you are eating in *My Fitness Pal* or something like it you will find a screen that lists all of your nutritional requirements and FDA recommended daily values. Notice which nutrients you are deficient in, and if you can incorporate those into your diet. If you cannot, supplement deficiencies with vitamins. Purchase the best supplements within your means. It has been our experience that Puritans Pride has excellent value and quality. Let us say here, that no product that we have named specifically is compensating us in any way. We are mentioning actual things that we have used and have found to be helpful. There are other brands, devices, and apps that are just as good if not better.

In the world of vitamins, and herbal supplements there are many options. As always you should consult a doctor or a healthcare professional. There are vast amounts of knowledge and opinions on the internet. If you are uninsured, or cannot afford to go to the doctor, supplements and vitamins can be a very helpful preventative measure for overall health and well being. You can get quality herbal supplements on the internet, in pharmacies, grocery stores, organic food stores, and holistic health centers to name a few. Often big chain pharmacies have free clinics where you can consult a healthcare professional. Organic Grocery stores and holistic healing centers often have resident herbalists. From our personal experience these people have been extremely helpful, knowledgeable, and friendly. They are not trying to sell you things you do not need. Most importantly they genuinely care about your health and the health of the whole community. We have yet to meet the herbalist that went into the profession to make a fortune. In our neighborhood we are lucky enough to have an holistic pharmacy. These people are the perfect blend of traditional pharmacology and new age holistic healing. They even make custom supplements for you. That way you can have your own customized blend.

When these four pillars of the program are put into use they will improve your health and immunity. For our purposes though this is just the beginning. So far we have not told you anything that is crazy or far out. We have not told you anything that you have not heard before. In the next chapter that might change. When we first found out about it not that long ago it seemed insane. We did our research and weighed out the pros and cons. The possible rewards of this home therapy greatly outweighed the dangers for us. We were amazed to find out that something that seems medically a little crazy and on the fringe could be so beneficial. We took the leap of faith and are thankful for it. We hope you take the leap of faith as well because this is the step that really protects you and makes you feel years younger.

7. Preparing for the Plunge

This pillar is the heart of the program. If you can only perform one pillar, this would be the one to do. This is the only pillar that has more than one chapter dedicated to it. We know you want to jump ahead to the remedy and start right now. We ask however that you bear with us through the next few chapters. The fifth pillar of protection is oxygenating your body through the use of a few drops of food grade hydrogen peroxide in distilled water in very diluted amounts. **Never drink brown bottle H2O2, you need to procure food grade H2O2. That is the number one rule that needs to be followed for your safety.**

Hydrogen peroxide is defined by the free Online Oxford English Dictionary as: *"a colorless, viscous somewhat unstable liquid, H2O2, which can act as* an *oxidizing and bleaching agent, is usually prepared as an aqueous solution, and is used especially as an oxidizing and bleaching agent in the manufacture of peroxides and organic compounds, as a weak antiseptic, and(in concentrated form) as a rocket propellant."*

Oxygenating your body greatly increase your immunity to disease, virus, bacteria, fungus, and parasites. The oxygen cleanse is beneficial for the lungs, metabolism, regulating glucose, and improving the immunity. It will detoxify your whole system, while banishing past disease and infection. It will bring your cardiovascular health to a level that it has not seen since your more active youth. Not to mention the fact that it will clear your complexion and give you a healthy, radiant glow that a supermodel would kill for. All these wonderful things are just the tip of the iceberg when it comes to this safe, cost effective, and easy to do home therapy.

We have to warn you that over the years there has been great deal of controversy surrounding this therapy. One camp says it is the miracle cure that will cure all ailments. The other camp says that it could be dangerous and possibly cause harm. H2O2 is classified as a hazardous substance. It is a strong oxidizing agent and can be extremely corrosive in strong concentrations. This therapy does not use strong concentrations, actually it uses very diluted concentrations. Much lower than the well known brown bottle three percent solution. H2O2 is used in many places to purify the water that comes out of the tap. The U.S. uses chlorine to purify the tap water. Water that is purified with Chlorine is much more dangerous, containing many carcinogens, and can have many harmful side effects. Chlorine is deadly in large concentrations. Millions of people ingest tap water every day with no fear of the consequences. H2O2 is also used as an alternative to pasteurization of milk. While on one hand oxygen therapy is accepted in many countries worldwide, and many doctors are making literal miracles happen in their practices on a daily basis. On the other hand this therapy is ridiculed and scoffed at by the established medical community in many countries in the world. The United States is unfortunately one of these countries.

There are doctors currently claiming great success with the world's deadliest diseases such as Aids with H2O2 and other oxidative therapies. Yes, that is right, there are actual doctors practicing in the world right now that are claiming amazing results with patients who have full blown Aids in direct result of these therapies. Aids is a deadly virus that is very similar to the Ebola threat we are facing today. They even originate from the same part of the world. The main difference seems to be that Ebola can be spread through casual contact with infected body fluids, and that it can kill you a lot faster. On the positive side of Ebola there are people surviving. Maybe not as many as we would like right now, but a little hope goes a long way. There have been people who were infected during every Ebola outbreak that have survived and gone on to live fruitful blessed lives. Ebola is a Darwin type virus: the strong survive. Our job as world citizens is to make sure we are as strong as possible so we can continue to contribute to this wonderful burgeoning world civilization, and assure its survival. Our theory is that if these therapies help with AIDS it would make sense that they would also help with Ebola. Our understanding is that it is the immune system that beats all viruses. Not drugs.

How will food grade H2O2 protect me from Ebola, along with other viral, bacterial, and toxic threats? H2O2 heals, and detoxifies our cells, which in turn improves the cell's natural oxidative properties. This means that our bodies will be able to use more of the oxygen that is available. White blood cells produce H2O2 to protect us from pathogens and other harmful things. H2O2 therapy benefits the metabolism and the digestive system. The digestive system plays a crucial role in your overall immunity. H2O2 therapy has been shown to increase the production of interferon and other cytokines that protect us from viral assault. The free online Oxford English dictionary defines interferon as: *"a protein released by an animal cell, usually in response to the entry of a virus, which has the property of inhibiting further development of viruses of any kind in the animal (or others of the same species). "* Cytokine is defined by the free online Oxford English Dictionary as: *"any of a varied group of small proteins which are secreted by cells of many types and which mediate cellular interaction in immune and inflammatory responses, cell proliferation and differentiation and various other processes. "* The immune system is made of cells, tissue, and organs. This system works to fight infections and keep us at optimum health. Interferon is one of the proteins known as cytokines which are messengers that signal the immune system to annihilate pathogens. There are three types of interferons. Interferon type I binds to cell surface receptors. Interferon type II is induced by cytokines as part of the immune process. Interferon type III is extremely important in fighting viral infections. Interferon signals other cells to join the fight. Interferon also literally interferes with harmful cell growth and multiplication. Interferon is vital to our immunity because it boosts the system's ability to identify harmful invaders. Interferon is the body's smart weapon in the arsenal of our immunity army. The body produces interferon hours after a viral infection. It takes the immune system many days to produce antibodies, interferon is the first line of defense. Interferon type I and III are activated once they have identified a viral threat. Interferon type II is activated by cytokines that deal with immune cells like T cells. Your body's ability to produce interferon is crucial when combating a deadly virus. Many viruses are resistant to Interferon; namely Japanese Encephalitis, Dengue type II virus, and Herpes. Furthermore, viral proteins like Epstein-Barr Virus, Human Papilloma Virus, and Ebola have the ability to inhibit communication between cells. The bird flu is very resistant to interferon. That is why having a strong immune system that has the ability to communicate is so important.

Hydrogen peroxide boosts the immune system's ability to produce interferon and eventually antibodies. Cells produce Hydrogen peroxide to neutralize or sanitize viral and bacterial pathogens. When increasing the body's intake of hydrogen peroxide you are boosting your immune system in two critical ways. The first being that you are improving your immune response time by increasing cell health, the ability to increase cytokines, interferons, white blood cells, and antibodies. The second way is by boosting your cells' natural ability to produce $H2O2$ as part of the immune defense response. $H2O2$ sanitizes your blood while neutralizing and killing anaerobic viruses, bacteria, and fungi. $H2O2$ also decalcifies and detoxifies the blood. When $H2O2$ kills a viral or bacterial pathogen it creates antibodies right in the blood stream. The more times oxygen in your blood destroys anaerobic organisms the more antibodies it can create immediately.

. Food grade $H2O2$ is a safe, economical way to help your body produce interferon. $H2O2$ is attracted to free radicals, bacteria, viruses, parasites, fungi and even tumor cells. $H2O2$ destroys all these unwanted things through a natural oxidizing chemical reaction. These are the things that will protect you in the first place, and fight the infection if, God forbid, it ever does occur. The oxygen cleanse will turn your immune system into a strong, well trained, well equipped army. You want your army to stand at the ready and be prepared to destroy anything that threatens it. If things like Ebola, flesh eating bacteria, and disease are even remote threats then we want an army that is invincible.

We have been told our whole lives that many viruses are incurable. We cannot tell you the number of people that we have met through the years who have to deal with viral infections for the rest of their lives. The most prevalent and common being sexually transmitted diseases like herpes and Human Papilloma Virus. These poor people have to deal with their infection and then worry about not giving it to anyone else. What a horrible way to live. We are here to tell you that there is hope. There is hope to get rid of past afflictions and there is definitely hope to protect yourself against future infections. Since going on the oxygen cleanse the two of us do not get sick any more. At work we have witnessed far too often someone coming down with something and before you know it four or five people have it. This seems to be an ever repeating cycle, every few weeks it begins again. These poor people cannot be happy because they are always sick, tired, and feel horrible. How many days have you called out sick in the last two years? We venture that if it is more than zero you have a compromised immune system. The first four pillars of the program increase your immunity greatly, but this fifth pillar is going to give you super health and super immunity. It takes commitment to see the whole course through. It is not the sort of thing you can start and stop. This remedy also requires that you use extreme caution and your best judgment. This therapy is quite controversial. There is a multitude of information for free on the internet, and many books on this subject. As always we urge you to do the proper research, consult a medical professional, and make your choice whether you want to do it or not. This is a jump start guide that is a call to action to protect yourself. We expect you to do your own research and make your own decisions and not just do something because we told you to. That being said you are going to feel the best that you ever have.

8. A Brief History of H2O2

Whole books are written that delve in depth into hydrogen peroxide therapy, its history, and the science behind the home therapy. This is a brief compilation of facts, medical studies, medical journal articles that we found interesting.

- In 1818 the French Chemist Louis Jacques Thenard (1777-1857) added dilute acids to barium and discovered Hydrogen peroxide.

- In 1863 the presence of Hydrogen Peroxide was proved to be found in rainwater collected during thunderstorms.

- 1888, the Physician I.N. Love publishes "**Peroxide of Hydrogen**" in the Journal of the American Medical Association, march 3rd,1888. In which he stated:

"After a six months' trial of the peroxide of hydrogen, considering the nature of the agent and its effect upon purulent matter and bacteria, I feel justified in concluding the peroxide of hydrogen is a most efficient means of cleansing purulent surfaces, deep cavities and sinuses, and stimulating the healing process in ulcerating parts. As a destroyer of microbes it is of great value as a local application in diphtheria and scarlet fever, ozaena, coryza and whooping cough."

The article below which was written in 1901 was found in the Massachusetts Medical Journal on page 411 of the compilation . You can find a copy of a compilation of articles written for the journal that some lovely person has made into a Google e book available on Google books just search for the Massachusetts Medical Journal 1901.

"VICARIOUS ABSORPTION OF OXYGEN IN PULMONARY OBSTRUCTION. *Insufficient oxygenation due chiefly to pulmonary obstruction is one of the gravest pathological phenomena, and to find a method to supply the blood with oxygen when the lungs are unable to do so is a problem indeed worthy of investigation. Practically the three most important diseases in which obstruction to the ingress of air and the absorption of the oxygen from it occurs, are laryngeal diphtheria, broncho-pneumonia in children, and double pneumonia in adults, states Dr. P. E. Doolittle. In the first disease we can fortunately make use of intubation and tracheotomy, and it is therefore to a consideration of the two last-named diseases that the author devotes his attention. The most available remedy for the purpose seems to be Marchand's hydrogen dioxide, H./3.,* which, as is well known, is chemically water with an extra atom of loosely combined oxygen. By weight this loosely combined oxygen is equal to about \ the weight of the hydrogen dioxide (more exactly, 1") and as it is in the nascent state when given off, it is much more* *active than the ordinary oxygen and is readily absorbed by the mucous surfaces, finding its way directly into the tissues. The medicinal solution of hydrogen dioxide contains 3 per cent, of absolute H2O2, and is capable of yielding 15 volumes of oxygen. This solution the author considers too strong and he dilutes it with 4 volumes of water before administering. The first case in which he tried the dioxide was an infant three months old, suffering with broncho-pneumonia. The disease was going rapidly to an apparently fatal issue; there was general cyanosis and every other evidence of insufficient oxygenation. A tea- spoonful of Marchand's hydrogen peroxide (diluted with 4 volumes of water) every five minutes was ordered, and this was continued for several hours. The breathing gradually became easier, the cyanosis gave place to redness, and the child recovered. The second case was a man of forty-two who had a severe attack of double pneumonia. Temperature, 104; pulse, 130; respiration, 56. Hydrogen peroxide (Marchand's) was administered freely by mouth and by rectum; eight hours after the temperature was 104; pulse. 120; respiration, 27. The disease lasted six or seven days and terminated by lysis, but the respirations never exceeded 30 per minute. Patient made a complete recovery. This case occurred in the mountains in British Columbia, where, the author states, pneumonia is especially fatal. Of the previous eight cases treated in the same private hospital, seven died. Of course, if desirable, oxygen may be given by inhalation at the same time, nor does the peroxide interfere with any other internal medication."*

- Dr. Otto Warburg (1883-1970)

was born in Freiburg, Baden Germany. He was a research scientist in 1931 he was awarded the Nobel prize for his[2]*"discovery of the nature and mode of action of the respiratory enzyme. He has shown, among other things, that cancerous cells can live and develop, even in the absence of oxygen.*"*
He deduced that Cancer cells and the tumors that formed where anaerobic organisms live and replicate by the process of fermentation in a state that is absent of oxygen.

[3]*"Cancer, above all other diseases, has countless secondary causes. But, even for cancer, there is only one prime cause. Summarized in a few words, the prime cause of cancer is the replacement of the respiration of oxygen in normal body cells by a fermentation of sugar. All normal body cells meet their energy needs by respiration of oxygen, whereas cancer cells meet their energy needs in great part by fermentation. All normal body cells are thus obligate aerobes, whereas all cancer cells are partial anaerobes. From the standpoint of the physics and chemistry of life this difference between normal and cancer cells is so great that one can scarcely picture a greater difference. Oxygen gas, the donor of energy in plants and animals is dethroned in the cancer cells and replaced by an energy yielding reaction of the lowest living forms, namely, a fermentation of glucose"*

[2] "Otto Warburg - Biographical". *Nobelprize.org.* Nobel Media AB 2014. Web. 5 Aug 2014.
[3] Otto warburg Nobel Prize acceptance speech *Nobelprize.org.* Nobel Media AB 2014. Web. 5 Aug 2014.

Make no mistake Dr. Warburg was a Nazi, he lived and worked under the protection of Hitler. His father was of Jewish descent but he was re classified officially as 25% Jew. He watched as colleagues where taken to the camps. He died in East Berlin in 1970. His work was used to do horrible things by a horrible government. Dr. Warburg was probably a very cold person. He never married, rarely commingled with anyone outside of his lab,and had close relationships only with horses. We in no way condone any of that. We want to look at his life giving work, we would like to acknowledge that his discoveries are the basis for Oxygen therapy. His most powerful theory was that cells switch to consuming sugar when oxygen is not available and thereby turn into diseased cancerous cells, and also that these glucose consuming cells cannot live in an oxygen rich environment. Dr. Warburg in his later years came to the conclusion that all illness came from pollution. In our twenty first century oxygen deprived high fructose centric world, we need to take a moment and stop and think about what we can do to help our bodies on the cellular level.We can collectively defeat disease and live in a state of ultimate health

- Dr. Edward Carl Rosenow (1875-1966)
Head of experimental biology for the Mayo foundation from 1914-1944. He published over three hundred medical papers. Thirty-eight of which appeared in the Journal of the American Medical Association. He believed that systemic diseases began

in the mouth.[4] *"Dr. Rosenow's investigations consistently
demonstrated the presence of specifically virulent
nonhemolytic streptococci within the oral focus, primarily in
or around teeth and/or tonsils (often without visible symptoms
of infection) ; these organisms or their derivatives were
directly and clearly implicated in a wide range of diseases -
from arthritis to schizophrenia and even including disease of
"blood- building tissues" The key to the success of Dr.
Rosenow's investigations was the use of a laboriously-
developed methodology that most significantly correctly
mimicked conditions existing within the human body,
particularly involving a range of oxygen supply, rather than
the customary reliance on strictly "anaerobic" (zero oxygen)
or "aerobic" (as in the air) conditions. The manner in which
Dr. Rosenow integrated and refined these concepts into an
understanding of a wide range of diseases may even come to
be recognized as the high point of 20th century medicine,
although his legacy is currently obscure or even maligned.
Surprisingly, this has occurred despite the association of Dr.
Rosenow with some of the most prominent names in American
medical history. Early in his career, Dr. Rosenow worked
closely with Frank Billings and Charles H. Mayo, both former
AMA Presidents and staunch advocates of the concept of oral
focal infection as a key factor in systemic disease."*

- In 1957 Dr. R.A. Holman published an article in Nature
  magazine, which is an interdisciplinary Medical Journal
  that has been published since 1869 it is the same

---

[4]by S. H. Shakman - Copyright 1996-8, all rights reserved.
www.instituteofscience.com

medical journal that was referenced in the beginning of this book.

"A Method of destroying a Malignant Rat Tumor in vivo*A hypothesis of tumour formation based on the catalase hydrogen peroxide mechanism in living cells was published recently[5] following observations on abnormalities occurring in aerobic and anaerobic bacteria due to certain respiratory irregularities[6]. If this hypothesis be correct, then a logical assumption is that agents which inactivate catalase or produce hydrogen peroxide (or free radicals) should have a detrimental effect on tumours.*
The treatment of experimental tumors with the catalase inhibitor sodium azide is effective[7]. Ionizing radiations have long been known to destroy malignant cells, and this may be explained as being due to the production in the presence of oxygen, in fluid systems in vivo, of hydrogen peroxide, the free powerful oxidizing radicals, HO2, HO, and atomic oxygen[8] as well as the destruction of the enzyme catalase.[9] Hydrogen peroxide has been given by daily intraperitoneal injections in animals carrying tumors without effect[10]. Makino and Tanaka,[11]however, observed temporary retardation of ascites sarcomas in rats on intraperitoneal injection of 1 ml of 2 per

[5]   Holman,R.A., Nature, 173, 424 (1956)

[6]Holman, R.A,., Lancet,ii 515 (1956)

[7]   Boyland, E. and Sargent,S Cancer Research,13, supp. 1,7 (1953)
Cudkowicz,G., Tumori, 40 63 (1954)

[8]   Bacq,Z.M. And Alexander, P., "Fundamentals of Radiobiology"
82 (Butterworths,London, 1955).

[9]   Foresberg,A., Nature, 159,308 (1947)

[10] Turner,F.C., Cancer Res., 18,supp. 1,81 (1953)

[11] Makino,S., and Tannaka,T., Gann,44 39 (1953)

*cent hydrogen peroxide and Hollcroft and Lorenz[12] noticed
some improvement of lymphoid tumors in mice after the
intravenous injection of hydrogen peroxide. Worrall[13] mentions
the use of peroxide forming compounds in animals and humans
in an attempt to set up catastrophic reactions in cancer cells.
It seemed to me that the only effective way to destroy the
malignant cells which are already deficient in catalase[14] and
sensitive to over-oxidation is to keep up a continued
administration of an active oxidizing agent. Since hydrogen
peroxide is an excellent ionizing solvent, and since it is formed
and is obviously of great fundamental importance in most
living cells, this agent appears to be the one of choice.
Rats implanted with the walker 256 adenocarcinoma were
treated by simply replacing their drinking water with dilute
solutions of commercial hydrogen-peroxide (Laporte
Chemicals, Ltd., London), and maintaining them on a normal
diet. The optimal concentration has been found to be 0.45
percent by weight and with the rats being housed in metal
cages (ten animals per cage) the rate of cure is on the average
50-60 per cent. The time taken for complete disappearance of
the tumour is usually 15-60 days. This of course, depends on
the size of the tumour when treatment is started. So far 72 rats
have been cured; they are now back on tap water and normal
diet, and will be maintained in this manner for the rest of their
natural lives. Ten of these rats have been cured for more than
two months; their condition is excellent and there is no sign of
recurrence of the tumor.*

---

[12] Hollcroft, J.W., and Lorenz,E., Proc. 2nd Nat. Cancer Conference., 582
     (1952)
[13] Worrall,R.L., Proc. Roy. Soc. Med., 49 (9), 665 (1956)
[14] Greenstein,J.P., Jenrette, W.V., and white,J., nat. Cancer inst,3,17(1941)

*This treatment has recently been used in four humans with very
advanced inoperable tumours. In two of the cases there has
been marked clinical improvement with decrease in size of the
liver,(which contained metastases)and progressive diminution
in the blood serum polysaccharide which Keyser[15]has shown to
be an indication of effective therapy in neoplastic states. A
detailed account of these experiments will be published
shortly.*

*R.A. Holman
Welsh National School of Medicine
Cardiff.
April 2.[16] "*

- R.A. Holman's findings were duplicated by a team of
  Polish scientist in 1958 as seen from the below letter to
  the Editors of "Nature" magazine

"**Experimental Chemotherapy of Tumours with Hydrogen
Peroxide** M. CHORĄŻY, A. GETTLICH, L. GÓRAL, B.
KOŁOCZEK, E. MOLAWKA, B. PENAR & Z.
SZWEDADepartment of Tumour Biology, Institute of
Oncology, Gliwice, Poland.

*"R. A. HOLMAN has reported1 that a high percentage of rats
bearing Walker carcinoma 256 were cured after drinking
hydrogen peroxide instead of water. These findings were not*

---

[15]   Kayser,J.W., Brit.J. Cancer, 3, 228 (1954)

[16]This article was transcribed from the PDF version that can be found at
foodgrade-hydrogenperoxide.com. It is referenced many times in the NIH
medpub database but sadly not available.

confirmed by Green and Westrop2, nor by Ghadially and Wiseman3 using Walker carcinoma 256 and Sheffield RD/3 sarcoma in rats. We have repeated Holman's experiment with some transplantable tumours of mice and rats.

    a. Holman, R. A. , *Nature*, **179**, 1033 (1957).
    b. Green, H. N. , and Westrop, J. W. , *Nature*, **181**, 128 (1958).
    c. Ghadially, F. N. , and Wiseman, G. , *Nature*, **181**, 1067 (1958).
    d. Schrek, B. , *Amer. J. Cancer*, **24**, 807 (1935).

• *Hydrogen peroxide (H2O2) is naturally produced in the body and is the body's main defense against infections. There is evidence that a common cause of immune deficiency may be a diminished ability to produce hydrogen peroxide. Hydrogen peroxide activates the body's white cells for a lasting boost in immunity and boosts mitochondrial function.*

• *A recent study by the National Institutes of Health (NIH) published in the September 2005 Proceeds of National Academy of Science entitled* ***Pharmacologic Ascorbic Acid Concentrations Selectively Kill Cancer Cells,*** *demonstrated that very large doses of intravenous vitamin C were harmless to normal cells and that the action of the vitamin C is as a pro-drug to deliver hydrogen peroxide to tissues (2). The authors conclude, "Taken together, these data indicate that ascorbate at concentrations achieved only by i.v.*

administration may be a pro-drug for formation of H2O2, and that blood can be a delivery system of the pro-drug to tissues. These findings give plausibility to i.v. ascorbic acid in cancer treatment, and have unexpected implications for treatment of infections where H2O2 may be beneficial (2)."

- *Hydrogen peroxide and large doses of vitamin C, and thus hydrogen peroxide, have been shown to improve natural killer cell activity*

- *A 1988 study published in the Journal of Advancement in Medicine entitled **Physiological and Biochemical Responses to Intravenous Hydrogen Peroxide in Man measured the metabolic effects of intravenous hydrogen peroxide in normal individuals.** The authors conclude, "We have demonstrated H2O2, when administered intravenously, has a pronounced effect to stimulate metabolic respiration... Intravenous and intra-arterial infusions of hydrogen peroxide (H2O2), reported since H2O2 kills bacteria, parasites, yeast, protozoa, inhibits virus and oxidizes immunocomplex (8)."*

- *A study published in Circulation entitled **Hydrogen Peroxide, an Endogenous Endothelium-Derived Hyperpolarizing Factor, Plays an important role in Coronary autoregulation in Vivo**, demonstrates that hydrogen peroxide is essential for the vasodilatation and autoregulation of arteries (10). This autoregulation has been demonstrated to be abnormal in CFS and very dilute intravenous hydrogen peroxide is a potential means of normalizing this abnormality (10,11,12).*

- *There is evidence that there is poor oxygen offloading to tissues in Chronic Fatigue Syndrome and Fibromyalgia that can result in relative tissue hypoxia and subsequent fatigue and pain. Oxidative therapies result in an increase in the red blood cell glycolysis rate. which leads to an increase in the amount of oxygen released to the tissues. There is a stimulation of the production of the enzymes which act as free radical scavengers and cell wall protectors: glutathione peroxidase, superoxide dismutase and catalase. They*
  > *activate the Krebs cycle by enhancing oxidative carboxylation of pyruvate, improving mitochondrial function and stimulating the production of ATP (8,13,14,15,16,17).*

- *A study published in Circulation entitled **Cardiac Resuscitation with Hydrogen Peroxide** demonstrate that successful resuscitation of a patient in V-fib, who was unresponsive to conventional resuscitation methods, was achieved with the use of intravenous dilute hydrogen peroxide.*

- *New research has shown that hydrogen peroxide protects neuronal tissue. This was analyzed in a study published in the 2005 Journal of Neuroscience Research entitled **Generation of Hydrogen Peroxide During Brief Oxygen-Glucose Deprivation Induces Preconditioning Neuronal Protection in Primary Cultured Neurons.** The authors state that "…hydrogen peroxide is likely the main trigger involve in the mechanism of IPC-induced neuronal protection (22)."*

- *In a study published in the 2005 Journal of Food Protection entitled **Inhibition of Staphylococcus aureus by Oleuropein Is Mediated by Hydrogen Peroxide** demonstrates that the effectiveness of the antimicrobial effect of olive leaf extract is via the production of hydrogen peroxide (23).*

- *Giving very dilute hydrogen peroxide (H2O2) is a very safe and effective treatment for CFS and FM.*

- *The safety and efficacy of dilute H2O2 has been published in numerous journals including The Lancet (24), Nature (25),Southern Medical Journal (26), Circulation(27), Annals of NY Academy of Sciences(28),American Journal of Cardiology (29)and American Journal of Surgery(30)andothers (5,16,24,31,32,33,34).*

- *Studies have shown these treatments are, in many ways, superior to antibiotics as well as being safer and without the problematic side effects of antibiotic treatment(5,8,16,24,31,32,33,34).*

- *The Study in the American Journal of Cardiology infused 0.2% hydrogen peroxide (over 5 times the concentration typically utilized to over 150 individuals without any ill effects. They conclude that …"H2O2 appears to be a safe, reliable and very effective agent (29)."*

*A study published in the American Journal of Surgery entitled **Use of Intra-arterial Hydrogen Peroxide to Promote Wound Healing** demonstrated that dilute hydrogen peroxide given intra-arterially could dramatically improve tissue healing (30).*

- *A study entitled **Influenzal Pneumonia: The intravenous Injection of Hydrogen Peroxide** published in The Lancet, demonstrated that intravenous hydrogen peroxide in 24 patients with severe influenza infection produced rapid improvement in a significant percentage of patients without any ill effects (24)*

- *A review of oxidative therapies was published in the 1996 International Journal of Biosocial Medicine Research. The author concludes, "This treatment had a cure rate of 98 to 100% in early and moderately advanced infections, and approximately 50% in terminally moribund patients. Healing was not limited to just bacterial infections, but also viral (acute polio), wounds, asthma, and arthritis.*

- *Recent German literature has demonstrated profound improvements in a number of biochemical and hematologic markers. There has never been reported any toxicity, side effects or injury except for occasional Herxheimer type reactions. As infections are failing to improve with the use of chemical treatment, this safe and effective treatment should be revisited (16)."*

*A study published in the 1983 Infection and Immunity entitled **Killing of Blood-Stage Murine Malaria Parasites by Hydrogen Peroxide** demonstrated the* *effectiveness of hydrogen peroxide in killing malaria. The authors state, "We now have evidence that hydrogen peroxide, which can also be released by macrophages, is effective against murine blood-stage malaria at concentrations which might occur naturally (32).*

- *Interferon treatment has been shown to result in significant improvement in CFS patients, but its cost and high incidence of side effects precludes its use as an effective treatment (35,36). hydrogen peroxide is a safe and natural way to improve natural interferon production (8,33).*

- *there was wide media coverage of a patient with multiple sclerosis that underwent treatment with intravenous hydrogen peroxide by a physician in South Carolina. The patient died several days after her latest intravenous H2O2 treatment and the pathologist erroneously stated the cause of death was a result of her treatment with hydrogen peroxide. This case was investigated by the South Carolina Medical Board and charges related to the use of intravenous hydrogen peroxide were dropped when it was determined that it did not cause or contribute to the patient's death. Rather, the death was a known side effect of the medications, Copaxone (glatiramer acetate) and Tegretol (carbamazepine), which she was using to treat her multiple sclerosis. This was the scenario specifically warned against by the FDA based*

*on post marketing surveillance. There are published
warnings by the FDA about the risks of long term use
of Copaxone and Tegretol which clearly state that they
can cause the complications in the exact same manner
and circumstances leading to the death in South
Carolina (41,42). On the other hand, there is no
potential for intravenous hydrogen peroxide to cause
any of the effects that resulted in her death.
Consequentially, the case against the use of
intravenous hydrogen peroxide was dropped.*

*Its unique broad-spectrum activity against viruses,
bacteria and yeast, make it ideally suited to the
treatment of these conditions.*

References:

*1. Walrand S et al. Specific and nonspecific immune response
to fasting and refeeding differ in healthy young adult and
elderly persons. Am J clin Nutr 2001;74:670-8.*

*2. Chen Q, Espey MG, Krishna MC, Mitchell JB, Corpe CP,
Buettner GR, Shacter E, Levine M. Pharmacologic ascorbic
acid concentrations selectively kill cancer cells: action as a
pro-drug to deliver hydrogen peroxide to tissues. Proc Natl
Acad Sci U S A. 2005 Sep 20;102(38):13604-9. Epub 2005 Sep
12.*

*3. Heuser et al. Enhancement of Natural Killer Cell Activity
and T and B Cell Function by Buffered Vitamin C in Patients
Exposed to Toxic Chemical: The role of Protein Kinase-C
Immun(1997)opharmacology and Immunotoxicology 19(3),
291-312*

4. *Vojdani A et al. Enhancement of Human Natural Killer Cytotoxic Activity by Vitamin C in Pure and Augmented Formulation. Journal of Nutritional & Environmental Medicine (1997) 7, 187-195.*
5. *Vesna Vujic´ a Stanislava Stanojevic´ b Mirjana Dimitrijevic´ Methionine-Enkephalin Stimulates Hydrogen Peroxide and Nitric Oxide Production in Rat Peritoneal Macrophages: Interaction of Ì, ‰ and Opioid Receptors.Neuroimmunomodulation 2004;11:392–403*

6. *Russell J M Lane, Michael C Barrett, David Woodrow, Jill Moss, Robert Fletcher, Leonard C Archard. Muscle fibre characteristics and lactate responses to exercise in chronic fatigue syndrome J Neurol Neurosurg Psychiatry 1998;64:362–367*
7. *Behan W. et al. Mitochondrial abnormalities in post viral fatigue syndrome. Acta Neuropathologica 1991;83:61-5.*
8. *Farr C. Physiological and Biochemical Responses to Intravenous Hydrogen peroxide in man. Journal of Advancement in Medicine 1988;1:113-129.*
9. *Munns SE; Lui JK; Arthur PG. Mitochondrial hydrogen peroxide production alters oxygen consumption in an oxygen-concen tration-dependent manner. Free Radic Biol Med 2005 Jun 15;38(12):1594-603*
10. *Yada et al. Hydrogen Peroxide, an Endogenous Endothelium Derived Hyperpolarizing Factor, Plays an important role in Coronary autoregulation in Vivo. Circulation 2003;107:1040-1045.*

11. Ichise M, Salit IE, Abbey SE, Chung DG, Gray B, Kirsh JC, Freedman M. Assessment of regional cerebral perfusion by 99Tcm-HMPAO SPECT in chronic fatigue syndrome. Nucl Med Commun. 1992 Oct;13(10):767-72.

12. Machale S et al. Cerebral perfusion in chronic fatigue syndrome and depression. The British Journal of Psychiatry (2000) 176: 550-556

13. Grahm J. Chronic Fatigue syndromes- A review. Journal of Australian College of Nutritional & Environmental Medicine Vol. 20 No. 2; August 2001: pages 19-28

14. Lindman R, Hagberg M, Bengtsson A, et al. Capillary structure and mitochondrial volume density in the trapezius muscle of Chronic Trapezius Myalgia, Fibromyalgia and healthy subjects. J Musculoskeletal Pain 3(3) 1995, 5-22.

15. Jeschonneck M, Grohmann G, Hein G, Sprott H. Abnormal microcirculation and temperature in skin above tender points in patients with fibromyalgia. Rheumatology (Oxford) 39(8), Aug, 2000, 917-21.

16. Rowen RJ. Ultraviolet Blood Irradiation Therapy (Photo-Oxidation) The Cure That Time Forgot. Int J. Biosocial Med Research Vol. 14(2) 115-32, 1996.

17. Frick, G., A Linke: Die Ultraviolet bestrahlung des Blutes, ihre Entwicklung und derzeitiger Stand., Zschr.arztl., Forth. 80, 1986

18. Finney JW et al. Protection of the Ischemic Heart with DMSO Alone or DMSO with Hydrogen Peroxide. Annals New York Academy of Sciences

19. Urschel HC et al. Cardiac Resuscitation with hydrogen peroxide. Circulation

20. Rowen RJ. Ultraviolet Blood Irradiation Therapy (Photo-Oxidation) The Cure That Time Forgot. Int J. Biosocial Med Research Vol. 14(2) 115-32, 1996.

21. Frick, G., A Linke: Die Ultraviolet bestrahlung des Blutes, ihre Entwicklung und derzeitiger Stand., Zschr.arztl., Forth. 80, 1986

22. Furuichi T et al. Generation of hydrogen Peroxide During brief Oxygen-Glucose deprivation Induces Preconditioning Neuronal Protection in Primary Cultured Neurons. Journal of Neuroscience research 2005:79:816-24.

23. Zanichelli D et al. Inhibition of Staphylococcus aureus by Oleuropein Is Mediated by Hydrogen Peroxide. Journal of Food Protection, Vol. 68, No. 7, 2005, Pages 1492-1496

24. Oliver, T. H., et al., Influenzal pneumonia: the intravenous injection of hydrogen peroxide, Lancet 1:432-433 (1920)).

25. Green HN, Westrop JW. Hydrogen peroxide and tumor therapy. Nature 1958;181:128-9

26. Mallams JT, Finney JW, Balla GA. The use of hydrogen peroxide as a source of oxygen in a regional intra-arterial infusion system. South Med J 1962;55:230-2.

27. Urschel HC, Finney JW, Morale AR, et al: Cardiac Resuscitation with Hydrogen Peroxide. Circ 1965; 31(suppl 11): 11 - 21.

28. Finney JW, Urschel HC, Balla GA, et al: Protection of the Ischemic Heart with DMSO alone or DMSO with Hydrogen Peroxide. Ann NY Acad Sci 1967; 151: 231 - 241

29. Gaffney F et al. Hydrogen Peroxide con trast Echocardiography. American Journal Cardiology 1983;52:607-9

30. Balla GA, Finney JW, Aronoff BL, et al: Use of Intravenous Hydrogen Peroxide to Promote Wound Healing. Am J Surg 1964: 108: 621 - 629.

31. Takeshita S et al. Intravenous immunoglobulin preparations promote apoptosis in lipopolysaccharide-stimulated neutrophils via an oxygen-dependent pathway in vitro. APMIS 2005:113:269-77.

32. Dockrell H et al. Killing of Blood-Stage Murine Malaria Parasites by Hydrogen Peroxide. Infection and Immunity 1983:39:456-459.

33. Tetsuo M et al. Induction of Interferon-gamma production by Human Natural Killer Cells Stimulated by Hydrogen Peroxide. Journal of Immunology 1985;134:2449-32.

34. Finney JW, Jay BE, Race GJ, et al: Removal of Cholesterol and Other Lipids from Experimental Animal and Human Atheromatous Arteries by Dilute Hydrogen Peroxide. Angiology 1966; 17: 223 – 228

35. See DM, Tilles JG.Immunol Invest. alpha-Interferon treatment of patients with chronic fatigue syndrome.1996 Jan-Mar;25(1-2):153-64.

36. Brook MG, Bannister BA, Weir WR. Interferon-alpha therapy for patients with chronic fatigue syndrome. J Infect Dis. 1993 Sep;168(3):791-2.

37. Lloyd A et al. A Double-blind, Placebo-controlled Trial of Intravenous Immungo bulin therapy I Patients with Chronic

Fatigue Syndrome. The American Journal of amed icnde;89:561-9.
38. Rowe K et al. Double-blind Randomized controlled Trial to Assess the Efficacy of Intravenous Gammaglobulin of the Management of Chronic Fatigue syndrome. J psychiatr Res 1997;31:133-45.
39. Takeshita S et al. Intravenous immunoglobulin preparations promote apoptosis in lipopolysaccharide-stimulated neutrophils via an oxygen-dependent pathway in vitro. APMIS 2005:113:269-77.
40. Wentworth P Jr, McDunn JE, Wentworth AD, Takeuchi C, Nieva J, Jones T, Bautista C, Ruedi JM, Gutierrez A, Janda KD, Babior BM, Eschenmoser A, Lerner RA. Evidence for antibody-catalyzed ozone formation in bacterial killing and inflammation. Science. 2002 Dec 13;298(5601):2143-4.
41. Medwatch: The FDA Medical Products Reporting Program COPAXONE (glatiramer acetate) Injection. July 6, 2000.
42. Physicians Desk Reference. Medical Economics Thomson Healthcare, 2005"

This cure might seem a bit over the top for some. We are not telling you to jump off of the cliff with us. We are leading you to the edge and asking you to take a look over the precipice. It is up to you to make an informed decision whether or not to jump. We are not advocating injecting yourself with hydrogen peroxide. If you feel that you need injections seek out a qualified medical professional.

What this cure has given us is unbelievable. Energy, vitality and a feeling of comfort because we know that we are moving towards perfect health and so can you. Anaerobic organisms cannot live in an oxygen rich environment it is time to blast away disease with the Oxygen cleanse and this is how you do it.

9. The H2O2 Protocol or the Oxygen Cleanse

Hydrogen peroxide(H_2O_2) is water (H_2O) with an extra atom of oxygen loosely attached to it that plays a vital role in both the health of our planet and the health of our bodies. Oxygen is nature's purifier. Dr. Rosenow had a theory that our bodies should be looked at as the physical world. That it is filled with different eco-systems that various diseases incubate and thrive in. Unhealthy cells and organisms cannot survive in an oxygen rich environment. That is why oxygenating your blood, tissue, and organs is so important. There are many oxygen therapies available ozone, hydrogen peroxide, Hyperbaric chamber, and breathing pure oxygen to name a few.

A proper diet that focuses on alkalizing the blood helps to oxygenate the body. Exercise helps to oxygenate the blood tremendously. The oxygen cleanse is the most affordable, and easiest to do. When added on to mind, diet, exercise, and supplementation you reach a whole new level of immunity. We have found it extremely safe.

Never use Hydrogen peroxide that comes in a brown bottle from the drugstore or supermarket. It will poison you because of the preservatives. **Only use food grade hydrogen peroxide that comes from a reputable source.** Call the holistic store before you go to make sure they have it. Double check with the herbalist or person in charge to make sure it is food grade H_2O_2 and find out what percentage it is. If you buy it online make sure it is food grade hydrogen peroxide and double check the percentage you are buying. There is a big difference between food grade 3% and food grade 35%.

Food Grade Hydrogen peroxide is a hazardous material and cannot be sent through the normal mail. If you buy food grade hydrogen peroxide on the internet and they do not charge you for hazardous materials shipping they are not selling the real thing. Always mark your food grade hydrogen peroxide so that you know what percent you are dealing with(important for safety). **Keep all hydrogen peroxide food grade and brown bottle away from children.** Always dilute food grade Hydrogen peroxide before drinking. **Never drink food grade hydrogen peroxide of any strength directly from a bottle.** Never consume food grade hydrogen peroxide in large concentrations. Food grade hydrogen peroxide is powerful, even though it seems pretty harmless, a little dab will do you. When using food grade hydrogen peroxide that is a higher concentration (12% or more) avoid contact with skin. Three percent is fine and is greatly beneficial for the skin. **Never get any type of hydrogen peroxide in the eyes. If this happens flush out with water, and contact a physician.** If concentrated hydrogen peroxide is accidentally consumed (three percent and above) drink massive amounts of water and get to an ER and or call a physician. When you go on the oxygen cleanse you are only putting in small amounts of food grade H2O2 into distilled water. **You always put your food grade H2O2 in with an eye dropper.** You can get eye dropper bottles at the pharmacy, or your organic grocery or holistic healing center. The most reputable companies on the internet almost always give you an eye dropper bottle for every bottle of food grade H2O2 you buy. We are talking about adding a couple drops to an eight ounce glass of distilled water. Even when the cleanse is at its most intense you are only consuming a very dilute amount. A little bit goes a very long way. As we neared the most intense part of the regime we doubled the amount of distilled water as a form of caution. **Always use distilled water with your food grade H2O2. Never use tap water, the chlorine in tap water will render the H2O2 inert.** Always consume food grade H2O2 on an empty stomach. Three hours after eating or one hour before eating. The main concern is that if there were harmful bacteria in your food the H2O2 would attack it, you would have a very upset stomach and feel quite nauseous. If this happens do not induce vomiting, that could cause aspiration of the H2O2 which could could lead to asphyxiation. We have taken it outside the recommended time due to tight schedules and have never experienced problems. We are all individuals and our bodies can react differently, so always use caution. There is a lot of information about this for free, so please do your research and find the food grade hydrogen peroxide protocol that is right for you. Our local organic market only had food grade 12 % H2O2 so we multiplied by three. That makes it the equivalent of 36%. The amounts added are so small however that we found the extra one percent made no difference.

This is the most common H2O2 home remedy. This is the one that is recommended in nearly every book or website. This particular regimen is attributed to Dr. David G. Williams. We have copied this from pure soul organics. A wonderfully informative website that also offers many free downloads on the subject. You find this by typing in H2O2 protocol, or Dr. David G. Williams to your search engine. The site address is 35h2o2.weebly.com. We added the 12% protocol. All of us have different levels of health and fitness this protocol is a general guideline. If you are suffering from serious conditions you may want to proceed as a slower pace. *"Food grade hydrogen peroxide is dispensed from an eyedropper into an eight ounce glass of distilled water. As the dose increases use more distilled water. Do this three times a day on an empty stomach.*

	35 %	*12 %*
Day 1	*3 drops*	*9 drops*
Day2	*4 drops*	*2 drops*
Day3	*5 drops*	*15 drops*
Day4	*6 drops*	*18 drops*
Day5	*7 drops*	*21 drops*
Day6	*8 drops*	*24 drops*
Day7	*9 drops*	*27 drops*
Day8	*10 drops*	*30 drops*
Day9	*12 drops*	*36 drops*
Day10	*14 drops*	*42 drops*
Day11	*16 drops*	*48 drops*
Day 12	*18 drops*	*56 drops*
Day13	*20 drops*	*62 drops*
Day14	*22 drops*	*68 drops*
Day 15	*24 drops*	*72 drops*
Day16	*25 drops*	*75 drops*

If you are healthy and doing this to cleanse, to oxygenate your blood, and ultimately protect yourself from disease then it is time to gradually decrease the dosage to a maintenance level.

25 drops 1 time a day every other day for 1 week.
25 drops 1 time a day every third day for 2 weeks.
25 drops 1 time a day every fourth day for 3 weeks.

*After that decrease dosage to a comfortable level. It only takes
a few drops consistently to keep yourself protected.*
*If you were not the perfect picture of health before you started,
and you are curing ailments with this protocol then you should
stay at the maximum dosage for one to three weeks. After that
decrease the dosage to twenty-five drops food grade 35
percent H2O2 two times a day for one to six months."*

Once you feel fully healed or you reach six months,
drop down to 25 drops one time a day for a week and then
gradually reduce the amount to a couple of drops a day or
every other day. To protect against things like Ebola and flesh
eating bacteria we recommend two drops per day.

This protocol is for adults only.

As the body is oxygenating and cleansing itself there
are times and ways that these toxins leave the body that are not
pleasant. Frequent urination, diarrhea, rashes, acne breakouts,
exhaustion, flu like symptoms, and mucus in the urine or stool.
These symptoms are the Jarvis-Herxheimer reaction and is the
effect of endotoxins produced by the death of pathogens and
other harmful organisms in the body. This reaction is also
simply called a

healing crisis. If it is ever too intense for you step back the dosage a day or two and then go forward. The fact that you are experiencing
this is proof that it is working. Stay well hydrated and focused on a healthy diet. These symptoms pass fairly quickly and are actually milestones on your journey to complete health.

Vitamin E will help your body use more of the oxygen that you have added. Also a probiotic like acidophilus, kefir, and kombucha. will help establish beneficial flora in the lower bowel. This will further increase immunity and boost the body's own production of H2O2. Later in the book we are going to show you
other natural ways of establishing this beneficial flora while getting many more benefits for your body and its immune system.

The following list is from an article published by Dr. David G. Williams the same Doctor whose protocol is listed above. We found it on Educate-yourself.org. He states that it is, *"a partial listing of conditions in which H2O2 therapy has been used successfully:Allergies, Headaches, Altitude Sickness, Herpes Simplex, Alzheimer's, Herpes Zoster, Anemia, HIV Infection, Arrhythmia, Influenza, Asthma, Insect Bites, Bacterial Infections, Liver Cirrhosis, Bronchitis, Lupus, Cancer, Multiple Sclerosis, Candida, Parasitic Infections, Cardiovascular Disease, Parkinson's Disease, Chronic Pain, Prostate Issues, Diabetes type II, Rheumatoid Arthritis, Cerebral Vascular disease, Periodontal Disease, Diabetic Gangrene, Shingles, Sinusitis, Digestion Problems, Sore Throat, Epstein-Barr infection, Ulcers, Emphysema, Viral Infections, Food Allergies, Warts, Fungal Infections, Yeast Infections, and gingivitis."*

Dr. David G. Williams claims that all these conditions have been successfully treated with H2O2 therapy. We figured with all this to gain and not much to lose why not give this protocol a try. We are glad we did. At this point we would like to share what our personal experiences were with the oxygen cleanse.

Once we learned about this H2O2 home remedy we thoroughly researched it and weighed out the pros and cons for ourselves, and then decided to do it. The next day we called up our local organic market and asked them if they carried food grade H2O2 . They told us that they did and so we rushed with excitement to buy some. To our disappointment they only had food grade 12% H2O2. We figured that if we multiplied the drops three
times we would be fine. The store also had brown tinted frontier medicine bottles and eyedropper lids for them. We purchased the food grade 12% H2O2, a frontier medicine bottle and an eyedropper lid for the bottle. All said and done less than twenty dollars. We rushed home to start the protocol. We then started day one which would have been three drops of 35% food grade H2O2, but for us it was nine drops of 12% food grade H2O2 in distilled water. First dose no problem. After the last dose that evening we experienced our first Jarvis-Herxheimer reaction(healing crisis) in the form of fatigue and flu like symptoms. It was uncomfortable and made us wonder what we got ourselves into. The next morning however we woke up feeling terrific. The most amazing thing was that we woke up without any pain. We are used to waking up sore because we were still recovering from our workouts, and daily lives from the previous day. That morning was different, no pain of any

kind, and actually feeling well rested. Not bad for immediate results. Throughout the rest of the day we felt wonderful. The most prominent thing being deeper stronger breaths than we had taken in years. All this and in just a day or two. As the first week progressed another thing became apparent, we no longer needed Ibuprofen, or any other pain medication to get through our workouts or our active days in general. Joint and muscle pain was something we had accepted as we got older. We always figured take a pill if the pain was to bad and get on with life. Neither of us has had anything but daily vitamin supplements since we started this protocol. The other pills that we stopped taking in the first week were over the counter allergy medications. For us seasonal allergies went away almost overnight. If the only thing this cleanse did was that we would still consider it a success. We also made a three percent food grade H2O2 concentration that we applied to our faces with cotton balls twice a day. Every couple of days we would put a few drops of food grade three percent H2O2 in our ears. Viral and bacterial infections love to hide in the ears. Ears play a big part in our immunity. As we progressed to the second week and higher doses things went splendidly. Cardiovascular wise we felt tremendously stronger and we were able to run farther and faster. We experienced an overall sense of well being and health. Our complexions became amazingly clear and people started to tell each of us that we had glowing complexions. Complete strangers would tell us how healthy we looked. Our resting heart rates had both dropped significantly in the second week. During that second week a good friend came to visit us right after a workout. As we were hanging out he could not believe how healthy we had become. He has known us for years and seen us at different levels of out of

shape. He noticed that we had lost weight, gained muscle tone, had a healthy vibrant glow. He even thought that J's hair was growing back and getting thicker. He jokingly referred to the concoction as wolverine juice. It is not named after the fictional superhero, but rather the sinewy beast that lives in the cold north and is feared by everything including bears and humans. That is actually how you start to feel, you feel like nothing can hurt you, no disease or illness can touch you. We have called it that ever since. As we started the third week and neared the maximum dosage we started to feel the healing and cleansing kicking in. Healing crisis became more frequent, but nothing serious. Mainly just a general malaise or fatigue. Some days diarrhea, and quite frequent urination. At times you could just feel the sickness, toxins, and calcification coming out of every pore not to mention every bowel movement. It was at this same time however that we both noticed that the other was not snoring anymore. we know many people, including one of us, who have spent a great deal of money attending sleep studies to deal with sleep apnea and snoring. We also know a great number of people who have spent a great deal of money on contraptions and remedies for snoring. Stopping our snoring alone was worth the twenty dollar start up cost. When we reached the maximum dose
we increased the amount of distilled water. We reached the maximum dose without any mishaps. We decided that for the maximum benefit we should go all the way, so we opted to stay on maximum strength for three weeks. That is 25 drops of 35% food grade H2O2 in distilled water three times a day. For us it was 75 drops of 12% food grade H2O2 three times a day. 75 drops from the dropper is quite a bit. One of the downsides of using 12% food grade H2O2 is the number of drops you have to use, it can be quite tedious, but trust us very rewarding. We

are not going to lie, the three weeks at maximum strength were very difficult to say the least. We experienced exhaustion, headaches, and irritability in the first week. These symptoms were not constant, they would disappear as quickly as they appeared. One night we would be irritable the next night fine. We noticed that while on the maximum dose our resting heart rates went up, but they were still lower than when we started. The second week of the full dosage was not as hard as the first had been. We still experienced healing crisis, but not as much. A day of diarrhea in the morning, a night of restlessness, or occasional exhaustion, these were the extant of the second week's downside. Something amazing was happening as well. You could feel it working inside you, different places, at different times. It never hurt or was in the least bit painful. It was almost as if you could feel the scrubbing bubbles of oxygen doing their work inside the body. We have to admit when you feel it working in your heart it can be a bit spooky, but so is heart disease. As the second week of full strength came to a close the cleanse became more intense. All the previous symptoms returned at different times plus another disturbing healing crisis. Mucus in the urine and bowel movements. It was not painful, just mildly disturbing. In the third week of maximum strength the detoxing seemed overwhelming at times. We actually took a break from our workouts in the third week just to let our bodies focus on healing, cleansing, purifying, and detoxifying. During this process when we experienced the worst healing crisis we still felt better than we did before we started. The benefits that we enjoyed up to this point were nothing short of miraculous, and definitely worth the different forms of healing crises. The downsides of this home remedy were

for us at least nothing more than minor annoyances. After the
three weeks at maximum strength we stepped down to the
maximum dose twice a day. Everything returns to normal fairly
quickly; actually at times you miss the third dose. We
considered this step a new start for everything. It was a time to
make a deeper commitment to our exercise and our diet. It was
time to burst forth with health and energy. That week we
ordered 35% H2O2 online from
WWW.pureh2o2forhealth.com. All said and done one gallon
of 35% H2O2 cost us $56.00 after hazardous materials
shipping and the discount code. The package arrived within
five days. We were both impressed with the speed of shipping
and the high quality of the product. It is so much easier to
dispense 25 drops as opposed to 75 drops. Once you have the
gallon of food grade 35 % you can make 3% solution to kill
bad bacteria and pathogens on food, and kitchen counters. We
made a large quantity of three percent and filled two spray
bottles that we bought from the Dollar Store. Always use
plastic spray bottles as H2O2 is an oxidant and will rust metal
in a shockingly short time. We use one bottle in the kitchen,
and the other for the bathroom. Always use caution when
handling 35% H2O2. We have found that it will sting your skin
and leave a spot that is pure white no matter your skin tone.
This bleaching goes away on light skin in about twenty
minutes, on darker skin it can take an hour or two. Neither of
us felt endangered at any time because we knew what to expect
and now you do as well. You would not believe how many
uses we have found for for the food grade three percent H2O2
dilution.

Some of the many uses we found

Kitchen counter cleaner/sanitizer
Bathroom cleaner/sanitizer,
Preserving organic dairy products
Vegetable cleaner/sanitizer
Poultry cleaner/sanitizer
Meat cleaner/sanitizer
Oxygen Facial 3%
Mouthwash 3%
Pre and apres shower mist
Sanitize and cleans dishwasher
Floor cleaner

Investing in the food grade 35% H2O2 was definitely worth the price. The gallon should almost be a year supply for the two of us.. There have been some instances of Jarvis-Herxheimer reactions, but not many. Any time either of us experiences any such reaction we see it for what it is. We have come to see healing crises as proof that we are still healing past illnesses. Throughout this process even when we felt our worst, we still felt better than we did before we started the cleanse. We know deep in our hearts that we are healthier, and our immune systems are much stronger than they have ever been before. Now that we are well on our way to completing this journey we know that it was worth it. This therapy has changed our lives for the better. We hope that you decide to join us on this part of the journey because we know that it will change your life as well. You will feel better than you have in a long time and any healing crisis encountered will be worth it.

The H2O2 Protocol

   We want to leave you with a few closing thoughts on H2O2. H202 is only one of the many oxidative remedies or cures. There are many other treatments available to you. Doctors can inject H202 into your system, or treat your blood with ozone and inject it back into your system. These are not medical mainstream practices; however there are doctors out there who specialize in these treatments. There are doctors in the U.S., but they are not easy to find, trust us. There is a lot of information about oxidative therapies and even lists available with doctors who practice these methods in books and for free on the internet. When we tried to contact the listed doctors for our area we found out quite quickly that the information on this list was inaccurate. We kept an open mind however and finally decided to do the oxygen cleanse. We are both very grateful that we did. Oxidative therapy, particularly internal injection of Hydrogen Peroxide is currently very popular in California. California is known for being a health conscious state, especially when it comes to holistic medicine. If you had to breathe the air that they have to breathe you would be very interested in holistic prevention as well. We liken the oxygen cleanse to when we added wheat grass into our lives back in the 1990's when we lived in Los Angeles. Wheat grass and the many benefits obtained from it were on the fringe back then. Now wheat grass is fairly mainstream and helping many people. There are many doctors outside the U.S. Who practice Oxidative therapy. Many Americans have sought out oxidative treatments in Europe and South America, and other parts of the world. If you are suffering from a life threatening disease we urge you to seek out a doctor who practices Ozone or H2O2 therapy. Many claim that the home remedy works amazingly

well on the conditions listed above as well as other conditions
that are not listed. After going through this remedy we agree
with them, the oxygen cleanse really is nature's miracle. There
are conditions, however, that need a more intense protocol.
One of these is emphysema. We have heard adding one ounce
35% food grade H_2O_2 to a gallon of chlorine free water in a
vaporizer can help with breathing. We have also heard that
internal injections of H_2O_2 administered by a physician are the
best way to go. Research your conditions, ailments, and and be
honest with the severity of them. Once you have done that,
decide what course of action is best for you. You after all, are
the only person in the world who is responsible for your health.
So make your decision wisely. We know that the oxygen
cleanse is the most important pillar of protection. We sincerely
hope that you work on positivity, diet, exercise, and
supplementation; They are all very important pillars. They
strengthen your body allowing you to attain the most benefit
from your oxygen cleanse. If you only change one thing in
your life as a result of this book, we both hope that it is the
addition of food grade H_2O_2 to your daily routine. It will raise
your level of immunity and protection. If you want to protect
yourself from Ebola and greatly increase your chances for
survival this is the quickest, cheapest, easiest way to do it. So
please as a responsible world citizen who wants to be
protected, join us on the incredible journey to perfect health by
way of the oxygen cleanse.

  The world population has reached seven billion souls.
That is an enormous amount of people for modern medicine to
care for. If ten percent of the world's population did the
oxygen cleanse, we would be a much healthier world. There
would be less burden on the world's medical systems because
minor illness would be a thing

of the past. Medicine could focus on the truly challenging problems such as Ebola and other highly infectious diseases.

If you would have told us ten months ago that our counters would be filled with colorful jars of fruits and veggies slowly rotting in water and a little sea salt, we would have thought that you were delusional. It is in fact true, it does exist and it is the 6th Pillar of the program. If we are going to be serious about health we are going to have to be free to talk about our digestive systems and elimination. To paraphrase the Dalai Lama, our highest function is to make excrement. We used to laugh at that little tidbit of wisdom. We did not understand that 85% of our immune system is housed in our digestive system. We always knew that it was an important part of maintaining and achieving overall health, but we did not realize the magnitude of the importance of our guts.

We have learned that the stomach is being looked at by Scientist as a second brain. 90% of the body's Serotonin is produced in the stomach. Serotonin is involved in certain neurological processes including sleep, depression and memory. We really must take stomach health as seriously as we do our mental health because we are learning that they are very dependent on each other. Did you know that your stomach actually sends[17]neurological impulses to your brain? What is it saying? Our guess is, "help me, I'm outnumbered down here there are 100,000 bacteria; please make sure that you are cultivating the beneficial bacteria, that I have a symbiotic relationship with." Thus enters fermented fruits and vegetables. They are superfoods that are packed with probiotics, very tasty, and quite easy to make. Probiotics are of course the good bacteria that promote the growth of the beneficial flora that we need in our bowels. Fermented foods are also thought to be

---

[17]http://www.scientificamerican.com/article/gut-second-brain/
Feb 12, 2010 |By Adam Hadhazy

natural chelators, meaning that they help to draw heavy metals out of your body so that they can be eliminated.

As with everything else do the best that you can, if you can afford to buy a fermenting crock, or any of the systems that are available for purchase please do so. If you cannot then a glass jar will work just as well. Let your imagination run wild. All that you need is a glass jar, distilled water, a little salt, and whatever fruit or veggies that you have in your fridge. Some people use Whey starters as they can then get a jump start on the fermentation process and save time. We prefer wild fermentation. It is easy, first you clean your vegetables and then cut them however you like; for example, grated, thick chunks, or any texture in between. Mix your ingredients and pack the jar as tightly as you can using hands that are of course very clean. One teaspoon of sea-salt per quart. Fill the jar that you have tightly packed with water, close, and leave on your kitchen counter until ready. Gasses will be produced inside the jars as the lacto-fermentation process is unfolding. Be sure to burp your jars to avoid excess pressure buildup, and moisture seepage. Make sure that water covers all of the food materials. Let stand from anywhere between two to fourteen days. Beware that it is a pungent pastime that you are embarking on, and that broccoli is an egregious offender. You are the judge of when it is done, taste it as you are burping it. That is one of the great things about fermenting you can really experiment. When you have a flavor profile that is acceptable to you simply put the jar in the fridge as that will slow the fermentation process to a crawl. Thereby allowing storage in the refrigerator for a prolonged amount of time.

Like any science experiment you will have great success, and at times you will wonder what was I thinking. We once tried a mixture of bok choy,seaweed,and carrots; to be honest that was a little too heavy duty for us. We have found that we really like making sauerkraut using green and red cabbages. We also enjoy fermented radishes, garlic, corn, and cauliflower. Fermented fruit not so much. We tried Apples,Pears, and Cherries and did not really like the saltiness of the fruit. It really is up to you, everyone has a different pallet, do not be afraid to explore and experiment. Below you will find the recipe for a simple beet salad that has become a staple side dish of our dinners and sometimes lunch too. This delicious and healthy recipe is scrumptious.

Beet Salad
Ingredients:
Fermented beets: about a half cup per serving finely chopped
Fermented green cabbage: ½ cup shredded
fermented radishes: 3 per serving coarsely chopped
Fermented Parsnips: ½ cup chopped finely
Fermented Garlic: 2-3 pieces finely chopped
Pickled Mushrooms: ¼ cup chopped
Blue Cheese: at your discretion

In a bowl combine all vegetable ingredients, mix and add in blue cheese. You can add a little balsamic vinegar and oil, or use balsamic salad dressing. We have tried it both ways and have come to the conclusion that it taste great if you use a dressing or if you choose not to.

Good luck on your fermentation journey, we hope that
you try it out. It is well worth the time spent doing it. We like
to think of fermented veggies as being a crossword puzzle for
our second brain... our stomach. Just like one should exercise
the mind one should also exercise the stomach. Do not let it get
lazy by consuming easy non-nourishing toxic fast or easy foods
prepared in a microwave oven. Connect with what you are
putting into your body and fuel it on a deeper more
meaningful level. We are eating mindfully, we have learned
how to prepare at least one of the right kinds of food that we
should be ingesting. That in its own right is very emotionally
satisfying. "Heal thyself," starts to make a little more sense.
There are many things that we can do for ourselves to make
sure that we are performing as optimally as possible and those
are the things that we should now be doing. We have to take
responsibility for the things that we stuff our faces with. All
Fast and Junk foods are loaded with addictive and harmful
preservatives and additives. Be strong and forgo those things;
they are poison and punishment foods. We love ourselves
enough to prepare and eat life giving true comfort foods.

11. Otolaryngological Health "Ear nose and throat cleanse"

The seventh pillar of protection is the Sinus and oral cleanse. The otolaryngological system plays a vital role in your immune system. The free online Oxford English dictionary defines otolaryngology as: *"The branch of medical science that deals with the ear nose and throat."* The ear, nose, and throat work together in harmony to protect us from pathogens, virus, bacteria, and other toxins. Even though Ebola is not an airborne virus, it has the ability to survive on surfaces. Contact with such surfaces could compromise the otolaryngological system. There are many other airborne viruses and bacteria that we are exposed to everyday; these could compromise our immune system right when we need it the most.

The amount of pollutants and toxins in the air today torment our immune systems. We as a world population are experiencing a great many allergies. People have always suffered allergies of one form or another. When you combine the modern diet with the current state of air quality in the world we are creating a recipe for disaster. How many people do you know who suffer from severe allergies? We are fairly sure that if you yourself do not have any allergies, that you at least know a couple people who do suffer them. Medical treatment from allergists and otolaryngologists will provide relief from allergies. Sinus and oral cleanses are beneficial for not only relief of allergic symptoms, but your overall health and immunity as well.

Nasal irrigation is also known as nasal lavage. It is the practice of flushing away excess mucus and debris from the sinus cavity and nose. There are many ways to cleanse or rinse the sinus, the one that we prefer is the Neti Pot. People have been using Neti Pots for millennia . It is one of the most tried and true home therapies available; therefore half of the seventh pillar of protection is the Neti Pot. The Neti Pot is very affordable and extremely safe when used properly. This is a home remedy that we have been using for about a decade now. We first heard of the Neti Pot about a decade prior to that. We had severe head colds and figured what could we lose, so we bought a Neti Pot along with all the other usual over the counter cold remedies. We were both impressed by the Neti Pot from the first use. We were convinced and still are to this day that the Neti Pot helps you rid your body of infection. Many colds and other infections have either been prevented or treated with the Neti Pot by us over the years. Neither of us has missed a day of work due to sickness in three years. Any time either of us has experienced even the slightest tickle in our throat or soft palate we turn to the Neti Pot immediately. The times when we have waited till the day after the symptoms appeared we have fallen ill. The times when we used the Neti Pot at the first sign of illness we have either averted infection or greatly reduced the time for recovery. We believe in the Neti Pot and consider it one of our most important weapons in our health arsenal. You need to use caution and follow the directions, but once you get comfortable with it, we are sure that you are going to love it.

Neti Pots are fairly new to Western culture. The benefits of this home therapy have only been known in the West for about a hundred years. In the east however the Neti Pot has been used since ancient times. The benefits of the Neti Pot have been known for many millennia in India. The discipline of yoga considers the

Neti Pot an essential tool for physical well being and spiritual enlightenment.

The first recorded use of the Neti Pot is in the ancient Hindu practice of Ayurveda. Neti translates to nasal irrigation in the language Sanskrit. It is believed that the Sanskrit language may have been spoken in India as early as the second millennium BCE. Scholars believe that the language migrated from the region around modern day Iran. The language was spoken long before it arrived in the region which is modern day India and Pakistan. People have been using the Neti Pot for a very long time. Hatha yoga employs the Neti Pot as part of the shatkarma, which is also known as as yogic body cleansing. The use of the Neti Pot is known as Jala Neti in hatha yoga. It is believed that clear nasal passages lead to clear thinking. The Neti Pot became more popular in the west during the late sixties and early seventies. People who went to seek enlightenment in India amongst the great Yogis brought the Neti Pot home with them. Slowly they grew in popularity and were considered a wonderful homeopathic practice. The Neti Pot became mainstream in the U.S. when Dr. Oz featured them on *Oprah.*

You can obtain a Neti Pot at almost any pharmacy or drugstore. They are also for sale online. Manufacturers include very important instructions, read them carefully. Neti Pots come in many shapes, sizes and colors. The most popular design looks like a cross between a miniature watering can and a magic lamp containing a genie. The only forms of magic associated with the Neti Pot are its cleansing and healing properties.

There are many benefits associated with the Neti Pot. The flushing of bacteria and dirt laden mucus from the nose. It helps with ear infections, and tinnitus. It can help alleviate asthma and bronchitis by clearing the nasal passageways. The Neti Pot is beneficial for eye health; it improves vision while clearing and brightening the eyes. It may help calm and soothe the brain and could help headaches, migraines, and even possibly epilepsy. The Neti Pot improves the senses of taste and smell. It can benefit the pituitary gland and balance hormones. It is believed by many that the Neti Pot brings clarity of mind, increases visualization, and improves meditation. This could definitely help all of us with the first pillar of positive mind. It is even thought by some that it could help moderate mood and behavioral disorders. We can both attest to the Neti Pot's effectiveness.

There are some risks with the Neti Pot, but those are nullified with responsible use. The FDA has issued a warning concerning Neti Pots. The warning states that improper use of Neti Pots could result in serious and even potentially fatal infections. The main safety precaution is the use of sterile water for the nasal rinse. Never use tap water, it could be harmful or fatal. Municipal tap water can have small amounts of bacteria, microorganisms, and protozoa. They are supposedly harmless to swallow. They could be potentially lethal in the nasal passages, because they could remain alive and cause serious illness. The whole point of this book is prevent illness, so please use distilled water, the purest sodium chloride available(never use iodized salt), and sterilize your neti pot with food grade H_2O_2 or food grade grain alcohol(Everclear). Always rinse and dry after sterilization. Never use iodized salt. Burning your nasal passage and sinus is a potential problem associated with improper Neti Pot use. You want to use warm water, but if the water is too hot it could scald or burn you inside your nasal passage. That would be disastrous, so please use warm distilled water for your safety. Cool or cold water is also uncomfortable, but it will not injure you like hot water. We have experienced water that was just a little too hot. Neither of us were injured, but it was far from comfortable. We experienced fairly intense pain and profuse watering from the eyes. Trust us, better to be lukewarm and safe than have scalding water run through the inside of your head. We advise you to follow the manufacturers instruction and heed the FDA warning about tap water. Through proper use the cleansing and healing that takes place is wondrous.

Here is our personal guide for Neti Pot use. There are two ways to use the Neti Pot:

- The first is the method most people use, where you pour the warm distilled saline water solution in one nostril and let it flow through the other nostril. This is the easy way that anyone can do and eventually become comfortable with.

- The second way is a technique used by yogis. This is where you pour the water into your nostril and let it flow through your soft palate and out your mouth. It is uncomfortable at first, and can be quite hard to perform. The benefits however are better than the aforementioned method.

The first method is quite easy. Use lukewarm to warm
distilled water, and a little unprocessed pure organic salt (never
use iodized salt). Never use water that is too warm, it could
damage the soft tissues of the nasal passages. Salinity depends
on personal preference, we advise you to start with a fairly low
salt level and work your way up to the salinity level that you
prefer. Mix the solution very well, make sure that all the salt
has dissolved and is not sitting on the bottom of your Neti Pot.
We usually stir about 50 quick rotations reversing direction at
irregular intervals. Lean over your bathroom sink and tilt your
head to the right, less than ninety degrees, but almost there.
Pour the warm distilled saline solution into your left nostril and
let it flow out of your right nostril into the sink. Gently blow
both nostrils into the sink basin. After that blow your nose
gently into a tissue a couple of times. Repeat the entire process
on the other side. Always clean and sterilize/sanitize the sink
when you are finished. Always clean, sterilize/sanitize, and
completely dry your Neti Pot after each use, so it is ready for
the next use.

The second method is the one that is in use by Yogis. It
is more complex and difficult to fully master. Never do this
one while you are alone. Always have someone spot you in
case you start to choke or asphyxiate. Just getting a little water
through the soft palate could have tremendous benefits. Mix
the same lukewarm distilled saline solution (never use iodized
salt). Mix just like the first time, about 50 brisk stirs reversing
direction every once in a while. This time you are going to tilt
your head back so that you are looking up at the ceiling. Close
your right nostril with your right index finger. Gently insert the
Neti Pot spout in your left nostril with your left hand. Relax
and see if the water will naturally flow down through your soft
palate and into your mouth. If this does not happen naturally

we suggest giving a couple gentle snorts. Once you feel water entering your mouth lean forward and spit it out into the sink. Be careful not to aspirate the water as that could cause asphyxiation. If some solution does go down your throat or the wrong pipe, cough it up immediately. The chance of this happening is why we say always have someone there to help you in case you need it. They need to be watching you, because if you do start to choke you might not be able to communicate verbally with your spotter. Once you are satisfied that the first nostril is done it is time to repeat this whole process on the other side.

Since starting the Oxygen Cleanse we have experimented with putting food grade hydrogen peroxide in our Neti Pot. A little food grade hydrogen peroxide goes a long way. From our experience one drop of food grade 35% H2O2 is quite adequate. If you are using food grade 12% H2O2 we recommend no more than two drops. These recommendations are based on our own experiences with different amounts of drops and different percentages. A little food grade three percent H2O2 is probably the safest way to go. There is debate over H2O2 in the nasal passageways. Some people believe it is wonderful, while others believe it could be detrimental. We do not put Food Grade H2O2 in every time we use the Neti Pot. We add a drop very sparingly every once in a while. We have never experienced ill side effects. What we are comfortable with and works for us, might not be the right option for you. You know yourself and what you can handle better than anyone else. That is the first half of the seventh pillar, next is the Oral Cleanse.

The Oral Cleanse is the simplest of all the methods discussed in this book. It will cleanse bacteria, toxins, and viruses out of your throat while making your gums healthy, your teeth white, and breath fresh. It will also clear out the harmful streptococci from the mouth and tonsil area. Remember Dr. Rosenow and his discoveries that harmful streptococci in the oral cavity are the cause of mental disorders, arthritis, along with a myriad of other conditions. He identified 35 different forms of streptococci that live in our oral cavity. Let us gargle them away. It is similar to a salt water rinse and gargle, except that it is a food grade three percent or less H_2O_2 rinse and gargle. If you wanted you could add unprocessed, iodine free natural salt, but it is not necessary. Never swallow food grade three percent or more H_2O_2. If you do swallow food grade three percent H_2O_2 by accident drink copious amounts of water and contact a medical professional. As a rule treat it just like any other mouthwash, you would not want to drink that either. After flossing, but before brushing take a small amount of Food grade three percent or less H_2O_2 into your mouth just like normal mouthwash. Swish it around in your mouth over your teeth and gums. Then tilt your head back and gargle for a good long time. Spit about half the liquid out and repeat the process with the remaining half. You will notice that it foams up. That is because the H_2O_2 has been activated in the process of sanitizing your oral cavity. Spit everything out and then rinse and gargle with regular water. The chlorine in tap water will deactivate the H_2O_2 in the oral cleanse.

The FDA approves the use of Brown bottle three percent H2O2 as an oral debriding agent. We believe that food grade
H2O2 is a much safer option. Brown bottle, while approved by the FDA for this purpose, contains preservatives and chemicals that can be extremely harmful to you. Food grade three percent H2O2 is a superior option.

So now you are working on positive mindfulness, exercise, diet, supplementation, drinking wolverine juice, eating fermented veggies, and cleansing your otolaryngological system. Your immune system has become quite strong, it is now time to take it to the next level with the thousand year old elixir which is the eighth pillar. This will give your immunity the strength it needs to defeat whatever foes that threaten it.

12. Beet Kvass

For well over a millennium the people of Russia,Ukraine and other Slavic states have enjoyed an amazing life affirming beverage that is known as Kvass. Tolstoy felt the need to mention it in not only one but three novels: *Anna Karenina, War and Peace*, and *The Death of Ivan Ilyvich*. Dostoevsky has *Aloysha* the youngest son in *The Brothers Karamazov* living in a monastery that brews their own Kvass. Chekhov has *Lopakhin* the ex-serf that ends up owning the estate mention kvass very early in *The Cherry Orchard*. If three of the greatest literary minds of all time thought enough of kvass to mention it then of course we can give it its own chapter. It is in fact the eighth pillar of our Ebola and all other infectious disease busting manifesto. Made from just beetroot, water and salt. This pillar is just as important as the oxygen cleanse! Beet Kvass is a simple yet potent additive to our wellness arsenal. Beets are a superfood, they have been studied extensively for their medically therapeutic properties. Beets are full of nitrates, which assist in the production of nitric oxide. Nitric oxide widens and relaxes blood vessels which leads to lower blood pressure. This is what WebMD says about nitrates, *"Nitrates also dilate veins throughout the body so that they can hold more blood. This reduces the amount of blood going back to the heart, reducing the heart's workload."*

In 2010 a study was performed at Queen Mary University of London in which it was shown that: *"beetroot and nitrate capsules are equally effective in lowering blood pressure indicating that it is the nitrate content of beetroot juice that underlies its potential to reduce blood pressure. We also found that only a small amount of juice is needed – just 250ml - to have this effect, and that the higher the blood pressure at the start of the study the greater the decrease caused by the nitrate."* The above quoted article was published in the American Heart Association online journal *Hypertension.*

Beet Kvass is used in cancer therapy throughout Europe and is frequently recommended to cancer patients undergoing radiation therapy . Beet Kvass is also a good source of natural iodine. Iodine is an essential trace element. The Encyclopedia Britannica defines a trace element as follows:

*"a **trace element,** also called Micro nutrient, in biology, any chemical element required by living organisms in minute amounts, usually as part of a vital enzyme, a cell-produced catalytic protein. Exact needs vary among species, but commonly required plant micronutrients include copper, boron, zinc, manganese, and molybdenum. Animals also require manganese, iodine, and cobalt. Lack of a necessary plant micronutrient in the soil causes plant deficiency diseases; lack of animal micronutrients in the soil may not harm the plants, but, without them, animals feeding solely on those plants develop deficiency diseases."*

Beets are also packed full of Potassium, Magnesium, and many other vital nutrients. They also have Betacyanin Which has been shown in studies to slow cancerous growths in prostate and breast cancer cells. Below is a fascinating study done by the Department of Pharmaceutical Sciences, Howard University, Washington, DC 20059, USA. gkapadia@howard.edu:

"Cytotoxic effect of the red beetroot (Beta vulgaris L.) extract compared to doxorubicin (Adriamycin) in the human prostate (PC-3) and breast (MCF-7) cancer cell lines.

Previous cancer chemoprevention studies from our laboratories and by other investigators have demonstrated that the extract of red beetroot (Beta vulgaris L.), the FDA approved red food color E162, can be effective in suppressing the development of multi-organ tumors in experimental animals. To further explore this finding, we have compared the cytotoxic effect of the red beetroot extract with anticancer drug, doxorubicin (adriamycin) in the androgen-independent human prostate cancer cells (PC-3) and in the well-established estrogen receptor-positive human breast cancer cells (MCF-7). This red colored anticancer antibiotic was selected for comparative cytotoxic study because its chemical structure with a planar configuration of an aromatic chromophore attached to a sugar molecule is remarkably similar to that of betanin, the beetroot extract constituent primarily responsible for its red color. Both doxorubicin and the beetroot extract exhibited a dose-dependent cytotoxic effect in the two cancer cell lines tested. Although the cytotoxicity of the beetroot extract was significantly lower when compared to doxorubicin, it continued to decrease the growth rate of the PC-3 cells (3.7% in 3 days vs. 12.5% in 7 days) when tested at the concentration of 29 μg/ml. In contrast, doxorubicin, at the same concentration level, completely inhibited the growth of the PC-3 cells in three days. Similarly, comparative studies in the normal human skin FC and liver HC cell lines showed that the beetroot extract had significantly lower cytotoxic effect than doxorubicin (8.6% vs. 100%, respectively, at 29 μg/ml concentration of each, three-day test period). The results suggest that betanin, the major betacyanin constituent, may play an important role in the cytotoxicity exhibited by the red beetroot extract. Further studies are needed to evaluate the chemopreventive potentials of the beetroot extract when used alone or in combination with doxorubicin to mitigate the toxic side-effects of the later. " This study is available on pubmed which is the National Center for Biotechnology Information a division of the National Library of Medicine at the National Institutes of Health. http://www.ncbi.nlm.nih.gov/. There are a lot of really interesting papers and reviews of medical literature. It is a great source of information, as is the Mayo Clinic online library.

In 2013 a study from the University of Exeter in England showed that people who consumed beet juice increased their stamina by as much as sixteen percent. The abstract from the study was found on pubmed and is below:

"Beetroot juice and exercise: pharmacodynamic and dose-response relationships.

Wylie LJ1, Kelly J, Bailey SJ, Blackwell JR, Skiba PF, Winyard PG, Jeukendrup AE, Vanhatalo A, Jones AM.Author information
Sport and Health Sciences, College of Life and Environmental Sciences, University of Exeter, St. Luke's Campus, Exeter, United Kingdom.

Abstract

Dietary supplementation with beetroot juice (BR), containing approximately 5-8 mmol inorganic nitrate ($NO_3(-)$), increases plasma nitrite concentration ($[NO_2(-)]$), reduces blood pressure, and may positively influence the physiological responses to exercise. However, the dose-response relationship between the volume of BR ingested and the physiological *effects invoked has not been investigated. In a balanced crossover design, 10 healthy men ingested 70, 140, or 280 ml concentrated BR (containing 4.2, 8.4, and 16.8 mmol NO3(-), respectively) or no supplement to establish the effects of BR on resting plasma [NO3(-)] and [NO2(-)] over 24 h. Subsequently, on six separate occasions, 10 subjects completed moderate-intensity and severe-intensity cycle exercise tests, 2.5 h post ingestion of 70, 140, and 280 ml BR or NO3(-)-depleted BR as placebo (PL). Following acute BR ingestion, plasma [NO2(-)] increased in a dose-dependent manner, with the peak changes occurring at approximately 2-3 h. Compared with PL, 70 ml BR did not alter the physiological responses to exercise. However, 140 and 280 ml BR reduced the steady-state oxygen (O2) uptake during moderate-intensity exercise by 1.7% (P =0.06) and 3.0% (P < 0.05), whereas time-to-task failure was extended by 14% and 12% (both P < 0.05), respectively, compared with PL. The results indicate that whereas plasma [NO2(-)] and the O2 cost of moderate-intensity exercise are altered dose dependently with NO3(-)-rich BR, there is no additional improvement in exercise tolerance after ingesting BR containing 16.8 compared with 8.4 mmol NO3(-). These findings have important implications for the use of BR to enhance cardiovascular health and exercise performance in young adults. "*

Easy Beet Kvass

Fill the largest glass jar that you own half full with beets that have been scrubbed and peeled and chopped coarsely. We use a gallon glass jar that has a pour spout. Add a teaspoon of sea salt, or rock salt. Do not use iodized table salt. Fill the container with distilled water. Cover the top of jar, set on counter two- fourteen days. As with all fermentation you are the judge of when your Kvass is done. When it is, strain the contents into another glass container. Be sure to scoop out the white mold that will form on the surface. White mold is good it is actually the beneficial probiotics that we are looking for. If you notice black mold forming in the Kvass throw it out. As with all fermented foods brown or black mold is not to be ingested the foods are contaminated and have to be thrown out. Trial and error has taught us to remove any beets that start to float in the liquid. We have read that the beets can be reused to make another batch but we have not had much success with that method. We use fresh beets for every new batch of Kvass. Keep in mind that the flavor of your beverage will mellow out in the refrigerator. Kvass is a beautiful, salty, sour drink. We always save the used beets in another jar in the fridge they are great to have around and they have a ton of uses.

      The first time that we had Kvass we stared at our wine glasses that held six ounces of beet blood red liquid that was vaguely effervescent. In that moment the myth of the Vampire made perfect sense. It looks like blood with its velvety deep purple hue. The saltiness of it is reminiscent of blood as well. The people who drank it all the time probably looked great for their ages and lived for a very long time. Yeah, sounds like vampires to me. Our little joke as we sip our Kvass these days is that one will look at the other and put on the worst Dracula accent that you can imagine and ask "Do you want to live forever...? Drink Kvass." You feel how good it actually is for you, one has the sensation that the body is actually saying "Thank You" as you finish your glass.

13. Putting it all Together

Now that you have been introduced to the eight pillars of protection. The next step is to put them all into practice. This can be overwhelming, daunting and challenging to say the least. This book proposes a complete overhaul of your life style, this is not easy to implement. The chapters have revealed the steps to ultimate health and superior immunity, but only you can make the commitment to transform yourself. As humans we make commitments and break them constantly. We break commitments to others and worst of all we break commitments to ourselves. The obligations of life can often get in the way of commitments we have made to others or ourselves. When someone breaks a commitment to you it can be very disappointing, we all have experienced this a time or two in our lives. We have to learn to forgive people who break commitments to us and be empathetic to their situation. It can be even more disappointing when we break commitments to ourselves. We all have to learn to forgive ourselves when we break commitments to ourselves as well. On any great journey there will be times when the path is treacherous and you fall down in a moment of weakness. Forgive yourself and move on and pursue that commitment with even more passion when you start again. Try your best, when you fail, forgive yourself and move on. No matter how many times you fail repeat this process and you will reap the benefits of all the eight pillars of protection.

There is only one pillar that we urge you not to start and stop. That is the oxygen cleanse. If you make a commitment to the full cure you have to stick with it until it is done. The benefits of committing to the complete cure are nothing short of miraculous. There are currently thousands of people on this same protocol right now. There are currently thousands who are learning about it and considering it. Many of them are afraid to make the commitment, or are still undecided. There have been multitudes of people who have committed to this protocol or something like it over the past hundred years or so. There are many testimonials from these people praising food grade H2O2 and they consider it to be the ultimate miracle cure. It is a very difficult choice to make. Do you believe the people who praise this remedy or do you believe the people who say it could be harmful. Only you can make that choice and then commit. Once you do commit please stick with it. If you miss a dose here or there that is fine. Do not miss multiple days. Starting and stopping this regimen could greatly reduce all the benefits that could be realized by completing the entire course. Those benefits are healing past sickness, and preventing future illness and disease. Nothing in life is one hundred percent so give the oxygen cleanse the best chance it can have by completing the protocol. It is a seven month commitment to complete the full cleanse. Once you have completed it, you should never have to do it again. You can stay on a minimal dose to stay oxygenated, but you will never have to do it with such intensity ever again.

With all the other pillars do the best you can. We know that no one is perfect. There will be times when you miss workouts. There will be times when your meals lack nourishment. Sometimes you will give in to cravings. There will definitely be times when your mind and attitude will not be as positive as you would have hoped. As for supplements of course you will forget to take them at some point. All these things are understandable and completely fine. No one expects you to do the Neti Pot everyday. Do the best you can do to implement all these pillars into your life. Once you see how far a little effort goes with each of these pillars you will be amazed how much better your whole life has become. Once you start realizing the benefits of the eight pillars, you are going to want to make a deeper commitment to them as well as your overall health in general.

The basic premise is to start to control your mind in a positive way. The power of the mind and subconscious alone can completely protect you from all sickness and disease. It takes a great deal of work to master. It can take an entire lifetime to master the power of positivity. Then you start to work on your diet and develop healthy eating habits. At this point you start to add light exercise into your routine. After that you add supplements into your life. These four pillars are the foundation of the program. Do the best you can with all of them. Once you have a strong foundation then you begin to incorporate the other four pillars of protection to the best of your ability.

This book is concerned with improving your immunity. We want you to be healthier than you are right now. We know that human habits are hard to break and that our vices can be impossible to give up. Nowhere in this book have we asked anyone to stop smoking, drinking, or any other harmful habits. You already know that these actions are bad for you. There is nothing we can do or say to make you stop them, only you can do that. We want you to be mentally, spiritually, and physically as strong as you can be. Once you start to see the transformation in your life we hope that you gain the strength to address your vices.

We wish you all the success possible with this program. We know once this program has become a part of your life you will be a happier, healthier person. Once you have reaped the rewards of this program we hope that you can share it with other people. It is said that there are only six degrees of separation between all of humanity. When you start to experience the miracles that this program can produce, we ask you to share it with six people that are important to you. If we can all do this we can produce a mass wave of healing power across the world. The results will be astounding. We both dream of a happy, healthy world, where every human can achieve their dream in safety and peace. We know that getting as many people as possible on this program would be a good start to realizing our dream. Please join us on our crusade for ultimate health and happiness.

www.ingramcontent.com/pod-product-compliance
Lightning Source LLC
Chambersburg PA
CBHW070548290526
45790CB00002B/606